Practical Justice: Principles, Practice and Social Change

T0386592

This volume engages with questions of justice and equality, and how these can be achieved in modern society. It explores how theory and research can inform policy and practice to bring about real change in people's lives, helping readers understand and interrogate patterns and causes of inequality, while investigating how these might be remedied. Chapters outline ways in which theories of justice inform and are factored into effective actions, programmes and interventions.

The book includes an international selection of case studies. These range from global inequalities in development and health to cross-border conflict; from gender justice to disability violence; from child protection to disability-inclusive research; from illicit drug use to torture prevention; and from prison wellbeing to sexual and reproductive health and rights.

Together, contributors explore:

- how social science and humanities scholarship can lead to a better understanding of, and capacity to respond to, key social issues and problems
- the importance of normative reflection and a concern for principles of justice in pursuit of social change
- the importance of community voice and grassroots action in the pursuit of justice, equity and equality.

Envisioning a better world – in which concern for the just treatment of all trumps the pursuit of privilege and inequality – *Practical Justice: Principles, Practice and Social Change* will appeal to students and academics in disciplines as diverse as philosophy, political science, sociology, anthropology, geography and education, and in fields such as policy studies, criminology, healthcare, social work and social welfare.

Peter Aggleton has worked internationally on sexuality, gender, health and rights for over 30 years. He is an Emeritus Scientia Professor at UNSW Sydney, Australia; a distinguished honorary professor at the Australian

National University; an adjunct professor in the Australian Research Centre in Sex, Health and Society at La Trobe University, Australia; and an honorary professor in the Institute for Global Health at UCL in London.

Alex Broom is Scientia Professor of sociology in the Centre for Social Research in Health at UNSW Sydney, Australia. He is co-director of the Arts and Social Sciences Practical Justice Initiative and a recognised international leader in the sociology of health and illness. His current work aims to develop critical analyses of the social dynamics of cancer and palliative care, and the global challenge of antimicrobial resistance across contexts and cultures.

Jeremy Moss is a professor of political philosophy and co-director of the Arts and Social Sciences Practical Justice Initiative at UNSW Sydney, Australia. He is an international expert on climate justice. His current research interests include climate justice and the ethical issues associated with climate transitions.

Practical Justice: Principles, Practice and Social Change

Edited by
Peter Aggleton,
Alex Broom and
Jeremy Moss

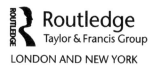

LONDON AND NEW YORK

First published 2019 by Routledge

2 Park Square, Milton Park, Abingdon, Oxon OX14 4RN
605 Third Avenue, New York, NY 10017

Routledge is an imprint of the Taylor & Francis Group, an informa business

First issued in paperback 2022

British Library Cataloguing-in-Publication Data
A catalogue record for this book is available from the British Library

Library of Congress Cataloging-in-Publication Data
Names: Aggleton, Peter, editor. | Broom, Alex, editor. | Moss, Jeremy, editor.
Title: Practical justice : principles, practice and social change / [edited by] Peter Aggleton, Alex Broom, Jeremy Moss.
Description: 1 Edition. | New York : Routledge, 2019. | Includes bibliographical references and index.
Identifiers: LCCN 2018056346| ISBN 9781138541658 (hardback) | ISBN 9781351010498 (e-book)
Subjects: LCSH: Social justice. | Equality. | Social change.
Classification: LCC HM671 .P73 2019 | DDC 303.3/72–dc23
LC record available at https://lccn.loc.gov/2018056346

ISBN: 978-1-138-54165-8 (hbk)
ISBN: 978-1-03-233850-7 (pbk)
DOI: 10.4324/9781351010498

Typeset in Baskerville
by Wearset Ltd, Boldon, Tyne and Wear

Contents

Contributors

Peter Aggleton has worked internationally on sexuality, gender, health and rights for over 30 years. He is an Emeritus Scientia Professor at UNSW Sydney, Australia; a distinguished honorary professor at the Australian National University; an adjunct professor in the Australian Research Centre in Sex, Health and Society at La Trobe University, Australia; and an honorary professor in the Institute for Global Health at UCL in London.

Alex Broom is Scientia Professor of sociology in the Centre for Social Research in Health at UNSW Sydney, Australia. He is co-director of the Arts and Social Sciences Practical Justice Initiative and is recognised as an international leader in the sociology of health and illness. His current work aims to develop critical analyses of the social dynamics of cancer and palliative care, and the global challenge of antimicrobial resistance across contexts and cultures.

Danielle Celermajer is a professor of sociology and social policy at the University of Sydney, Australia. Her research stands at the interface of theories exploring the multi-dimensional nature of injustice and the practice of human rights. She recently completed a European Union-funded multi-country project on the prevention of torture, focusing on everyday violence in the security sector.

Elaine Chase is an associate professor in education, health promotion and international development at the UCL Institute of Education in the UK. Her research focuses on the health and wellbeing outcomes of young people and communities, particularly those most likely to experience disadvantage and marginalisation.

Darryl Cronin works for the Edmund Rice Centre in Sydney, Australia. The centre promotes human rights, social justice and eco-justice through research, community education, advocacy and networking. Priority areas are Indigenous Australians and reconciliation, refugees and asylum seekers, and the impact of climate change on people in the

Pacific Islands. Darryl's research focuses on constitutionalism, democracy and justice for Indigenous people in Australia. He has over 20 years' experience working with Aboriginal organisations in northern Australia on land rights and socioeconomic development.

Assa Doron is an associate professor of anthropology in the College of Asia and the Pacific at the Australian National University. His fieldwork in India offers an ethnographic investigation of the state–society interface, focusing on issues surrounding the politics of identity, development, media and public health.

Leanne Dowse is a professor of disability studies in the Faculty of Arts and Social Sciences at UNSW Sydney, Australia. She leads a programme of interdisciplinary research in disability aimed at creating knowledge to build capacity to address issues for people with disability who experience complex intersectional disadvantage, with a particular focus on systemic responses to gender, indigeneity, violence and incarceration.

Karen R. Fisher is a professor within the Social Policy Research Centre at UNSW Sydney, Australia. Her research interests are in the organisation of social services in Australia and China, including disability and mental health community services, inclusive research and evaluation methodology, and social policy process.

Mel Getty is a founder, director and chief executive officer of the Aurora Project in London, UK, which provides a peer mentoring service for individuals in treatment for substance and alcohol use. Mel is a founding member of the Addiction Service User Research Group (SURG), which is supported by the National Institute for Health Research (NIHR) Biomedical Research Centre for Mental Health at South London and Maudsley NHS Foundation Trust and King's College London, UK.

Sofia Gruskin is a professor of law and preventive medicine at the University of Southern California, USA, where she serves as the director of the Institute for Global Health and its Program on Global Health and Human Rights. A pioneer in global health and human rights, her work, which ranges from global policy to the grassroots level, has been instrumental in developing the conceptual, methodological and empirical links between health and human rights, with a focus on HIV, sexual and reproductive health, health systems and more.

Lorraine Hansford is a researcher at the University of Exeter Medical School, UK. She has a professional background in delivering and evaluating youth and community work and in recent years has undertaken research in children and young people's mental health, health inequalities and mental distress, and moral narratives in low-income communities. She has a particular interest in engaged research, working alongside communities and community organisations at each stage of the research process, from design to impact.

Cassie Hogan is a member of the Addiction Service User Research Group (SURG), which is supported by the National Institute for Health Research (NIHR) Biomedical Research Centre for Mental Health at South London and Maudsley NHS Foundation Trust and King's College London, UK. She has worked as a counsellor in the addiction field and is a director of Create Recovery, which supports people with experience of addiction issues to develop their creativity. She is undertaking doctoral research exploring identity translation and recovery.

Max Hopwood is a research fellow in the Centre for Social Research in Health at UNSW Sydney, Australia. His research interests include the experience of living with chronic illness, particularly viral hepatitis and HIV, harm reduction, stigma, discrimination and the psychosocial dynamics of injecting and other illicit drug use.

Richard Hugman is a professor of social work at UNSW Sydney, Australia, and has previously taught, researched and practised in social work in Australia and the UK. He has written extensively about professional ethics, with a particular focus on social work.

Ilan Katz is a professor in the Social Policy Research Centre at UNSW Sydney, Australia. His research interests include the evaluation of complex interventions; the interface between research, policy and practice; child protection systems; children in out-of-home care; disability; Indigenous social policy; community, social inclusion and social capital; youth mental health; migration and asylum; race and ethnicity; and social policy in developing countries.

Rosemary Kayess is a senior research fellow in the Social Policy Research Centre and a visiting fellow in law at UNSW Sydney, Australia. She has extensive disability policy experience. She has held ministerial advisory roles with both the state and federal government on disability and carer issues and was the external expert on the Australian Government delegation to the United Nations negotiations for the Convention on the Rights of Persons with Disabilities.

Paul Lennon is a founder and trustee of the Aurora Project, London, UK, which provides a peer mentoring service for individuals in treatment for substance and alcohol use. He has represented service users locally and at a national level at Public Health England. He is also a founding member of the Addiction Service User Research Group (SURG), which is supported by the National Institute for Health Research (NIHR)

Biomedical Research Centre for Mental Health at South London and Maudsley NHS Foundation Trust and King's College London, UK.

Annie Madden is a doctoral candidate in the Centre for Social Research in Health at UNSW Sydney, Australia. Prior to this, she was CEO of the Australian Illicit and Injecting Drug Users League (AIVL), the peak national organisation in Australia representing people who use/have used illicit drugs. Annie is a co-founder and current board member of Harm Reduction Australia (HRA) and has a longstanding commitment to promoting justice and human rights for people who use/have used illicit drugs, and people in drug treatment.

Purnima Mane is a visiting professor in the Centre for Social Research in Health at UNSW Sydney. She has worked on HIV and sexual and reproductive health internationally and in India for over 25 years – in senior positions with the United Nations, non-profit organisations and academia. She is a board member of several organisations working within the fields of HIV and sexual and reproductive health and rights.

Leila Morsy is a senior lecturer in the College of Medicine and Public Health at Flinders University in Adelaide, Australia. Her primary research interest is the factors contributing to school achievement differences between African-American and white children. She has published on the effects of the family (including parenting and parent work schedules) and health on children's outcomes. Her work has been presented to educators, policymakers, physicians and the US Congressional Committee on Education and the Workforce.

Jeremy Moss is a professor of political philosophy and co-director of the Arts and Social Sciences Practical Justice Initiative at UNSW Sydney, Australia. His research interests include climate justice, the ethics of renewable energy as well as the ethical issues associated with climate transitions. He chaired the UNESCO working group on Climate Ethics and Energy Security, and has been a visitor at Oxford and McGill universities.

Joanne Neale is a professor of addictions qualitative research at the National Addiction Centre, King's College London, UK, and a conjoint professor in the Centre for Social Research in Health at UNSW Sydney, Australia. She undertakes qualitative, quantitative and mixed methods studies exploring topics relating to substance use, homelessness, treatment options and service provision. She is part-funded by the National Institute for Health Research (NIHR) Biomedical Research Centre for Mental Health at South London and Maudsley NHS Foundation Trust and King's College London, UK.

Alexandra Nicholson works in the Program on Global Health & Human Rights at the Institute for Global Health, University of Southern California. She has a background in social impact studies and social entrepreneurship, oversees the management and administration of research projects, and contributes to shaping and supporting the programme's research agenda, particularly in the area of sexual and reproductive health and rights.

Anne O'Brien is a professor of history in the School of Humanities and Languages UNSW Sydney, Australia. She has published widely in the histories of women, gender, welfare, religion and Indigenous policy. Her ongoing research, a history of homelessness and of people experiencing it, is being conducted with Heather Holst, the deputy chief executive officer of Launch Housing, and is funded by an Australian Research Council ARC Discovery Project grant.

Paul Patton is Scientia Professor of Philosophy at UNSW Sydney, Australia and a Fellow of the Australian Academy of the Humanities. He has published widely on continental and contemporary liberal political philosophy.

Felicity Thomas is a senior research fellow in the University of Exeter Medical School and the College of Humanities, and the director of the WHO Collaborating Centre on Culture and Health. Her work uses narrative, ethnographic and engaged approaches to understand how health inequalities are experienced, and to identify policy-relevant priorities for change. She has a particular interest in poverty and mental health, and how moral narratives and welfare reforms intersect to shape lived experience and healthcare responses.

Carla Treloar is Scientia Professor and Director of the Centre for Social Research in Health and the Social Policy Research Centre at UNSW Sydney, Australia. Her research encompasses the social aspects of drug use in relation to prevention of drug-related harms (particularly hepatitis C), the engagement of people who use drugs in health and other services, and the critical analysis of the structure and operation of services for people who use drugs.

kylie valentine is an associate professor and the deputy director of the Social Policy Research Centre at UNSW Sydney, Australia. Her research interests include the application of sociological methods and concepts to new areas and concerns, with a focus on social disadvantage and exclusion. She has conducted social research on human services organisation and delivery and on programmes for children and families. She has wide-ranging expertise in qualitative methodologies and evaluation design.

Acknowledgements

We thank UNSW Sydney for its support of the Arts and Social Sciences Practical Justice Initiative as part of which this book was developed. We are grateful to Tim Wong, who helped organise the seminars at which early versions of several chapters included here were given. We thank Sarah Hoile for liaising with contributors and for administrative and secretarial support.

Practical justice

By way of introduction

Peter Aggleton, Alex Broom and Jeremy Moss

Background

Over the last 50 years, in disciplines as diverse as philosophy, political science, sociology, anthropology, geography and education, and in fields such as policy studies, social work and social welfare, there has been growing concern with questions of fairness and equality. Until recently, much of this interest has been discipline-specific, with relatively few attempts made to develop genuinely cross- and inter-disciplinary understandings of the issues involved. Likewise, theory and research concerning inequality and exclusion often remain somewhat distant from the policy and practice interventions that might bring about real change in people's lives. In consequence, there exists a gap between those interested in understanding and interrogating the patterns and causes of inequality and those working to remedy matters through policies and practices that are socially just.

The idea of practical justice seeks to bridge some of these divides. Its origins are several but can be traced to philosophical debate concerning the just treatment of individuals and groups in society. Conceptions of distributive justice, historical or reparative justice, and justice as recognition have been central to this task. However, research within other disciplines – most notably sociology, human geography, social policy and development studies – also seeks to engage with questions of justice, equity and equality and the ways in which these desired states of being may be brought about. Work in fields such as social administration, human services, social welfare and social work also seeks to engage with these issues, by focusing on and prioritising the needs of some of the most disadvantaged members of society. But how best may this be done and how might socially just outcomes be achieved?

From principles to practice

It is within this context that the idea of practical justice has great appeal. This introductory book lays the groundwork for what must be thought about and done across fields and disciplines. With contributions from a diverse group of academics, academic–activists and scholar–practitioners, it seeks to identify a range of issues that any form of practical justice might engage with, and the outcomes that might be struggled for and achieved. A wide range of issues is focused upon – from global inequalities in health to cross-border migration; from gender justice to homelessness; from child protection to disability-inclusive research; from illicit drug use to torture prevention; and from prison wellbeing to sexual and reproductive health and rights. Across this diversity, authors are of one voice in their concern to demonstrate:

- how good-quality scholarship may lead to a better understanding of, and capacity to respond to, key social issues and problems
- the importance of normative reflection and a concern for a conception of justice in pursuit of social change
- the importance of community voice and grassroots action in the pursuit of justice, equity and equality.

The editors and authors have worked together over a period of 18 months to prepare the different contributions that make up the book. The focus of the chapters is intentionally diverse, to demonstrate the potential of a practical justice lens to bring about change in varied aspects of social life. Our goal has been to lay the foundations for future scholarship and research through contributions which, both individually and collectively, envision a better world – in which concern for the just treatment of all trumps the pursuit of privilege and the pursuit of inequality.

This book

The book is divided into two parts. The first of these aims to provide the reader with insight into how practical justice might best be understood, worked towards and achieved.

In the opening chapter of the book, Paul Patton and Jeremy Moss set the scene by reflecting on some of the most common approaches to justice in contemporary political philosophy: distributive justice, reparative justice, and a third approach that involves ensuring adequate recognition of particular peoples or groups within a population. In the process, they raise questions about what is meant by practical justice. Is it a distinct sphere of concern about justice or might it be better understood as referring to the issues that arise when we move beyond theory and theorisation to consider the requirements of justice in the real world?

In her chapter entitled ' "Homeless women": histories of emotion and justice', Anne O'Brien offers a historical perspective to understanding women's experiences of homelessness in Australia. Her analysis focuses on how homeless women were represented, and how they understood themselves, in the period leading up to the twentieth-century post-war welfare state. Through a close reading of historical evidence, O'Brien signals the emergence of different visions of justice and how, in the contemporary search for practical justice, the voices of structurally disadvantaged Others ought not just be heard but called upon to shape visibility and advocacy.

Similar themes emerge in Leanne Dowse's chapter entitled 'Worlds apart and still no closer to justice'. Arguing that recognition and redress are central to addressing gendered disability violence, the chapter focuses on the differential enactment of justice in contexts where gender, disability and violence intersect. Experience shows many women with disability excluded from processes of justice, while for others, intractable systemic enmeshment results. The experiences of two women, explored through case studies, reveals contradictory processes of exclusion and entrenchment that highlight the ambivalence of justice and its systems in engaging with questions of intersectionality.

Related issues emerge, albeit in a slightly different context, in Felicity Thomas and Lorraine Hansford's chapter, 'Supporting mental health in low-income communities'. This chapter points to the paradox between growing equity in mental health diagnoses and treatment and the discontent and injustice experienced by those living with poverty-related distress. The chapter identifies two inter-related ways in which forms of injustice impact on people in low-income communities: first, examining how experiences of poverty and engagement with the welfare system can exacerbate underlying vulnerabilities to mental health issues; and second, focusing on the wellbeing implications of medicalising poverty-related distress. Special attention is given to the relevance, effectiveness and ethics of current treatment options and their implications for more equitable systems of support.

Questions of injustice are taken further in Danielle Celermajer's chapter, 'Critical theories of justice and the practice of torture prevention'. Here, the focus is on the limitations of human rights approaches when it comes to addressing the structural underpinnings of injustice. Looking at the problem of systematic and everyday forms of torture, this chapter considers how critical theoretical approaches to injustice can be usefully taken up to assist in the practice of torture prevention.

In 'Poverty in rich countries: damage, difference, and possibilities for justice', kylie valentine considers how issues of poverty and inequality can be understood in analytic and normative terms: why do they happen, who should be held responsible, and what should be done to address them? The chapter focuses in particular on how best to approach questions of justice for those who may be seen as the 'undeserving' poor, in the form of individuals who seem to act against their best interests and resist attempts to address their needs. Within this context, the emphasis on trauma and the harms done by poverty, while valuable, can be risky. Recognition of agency and, in particular, desire may offer a more promising way forward.

The final chapter in this part is by Sofia Gruskin and Alexandra Nicholson. Entitled 'Engaging global institutions to achieve practical justice: the case of sexual rights', it examines how to progress issues of practical justice within the technical, legal and political streams in which global institutions work. Using sexual rights as an example, it shows how these different streams often move forward independently, while overlapping and drawing strength from one another to shape the current global landscape around sexual rights. Consideration of the interactions within and between these streams offers a useful approach to working with global institutions, with application to a range of issues relevant to practical justice work.

Part II of the book continues the task of linking conceptions of justice with practical concerns by focusing on a number of fields in which ideas concerning practical justice have had beneficial effect.

In the first chapter in this part, 'Practical justice in social work and social welfare: contested values', Richard Hugman looks at the question of competing values in social welfare and social work. The chapter examines how wider debates about social justice laid the foundations on which contemporary social work and social welfare stand. Central to social work and social welfare practice is the exercise of power, providing the basis for challenging social injustice but at the same time creating problems for how these very practices may or may not be socially just. The implications of these tensions are explored for efforts to eradicate poverty, disadvantage and other forms of social need.

In his chapter entitled 'A just child protection system – is it possible?', Ilan Katz engages with how child protection systems might work to promote the 'best interests' of children. Two major conceptualisations of child protection – the rescue model and the public health model – carry different implications for justice, but neither is satisfactory in practice. The chapter thus offers a framework in which the interests of children are balanced against those of parents, communities and society. With a focus on Indigenous and minority ethnic children, the chapter shows how just child protection systems are possible, but only if justice is viewed as an evolving rather than a fixed characteristic.

Different issues are examined in Karen R. Fisher and Rosemary Kayess's chapter, 'Collaborative disability-inclusive research and evaluation as a practical justice process'. Universities and colleges rarely make room for inclusive practice in research and teaching, despite their rhetoric about social justice and equity. One approach to correcting this injustice is through research that promotes inclusive practice. This chapter explores how partnership and close working with people with disabilities and the organisations that represent them can change research and heighten impact. Examples from research projects initiated by community partners or government illustrate how such an approach can modify the questions asked, the methods applied and the ways in which results are used.

In his chapter on 'Justice and the political future for Indigenous Australians', Darryl Cronin draws attention to the importance of resistance and political resurgence as a means to achieving justice. In recent decades, the rights-based claims of Aboriginal and Torres Strait Islander peoples have been systematically rejected by successive Australian governments, being substituted for by narratives of Indigenous dysfunction and socio-economic inequality. Political gains since the 1970s have been undone and Indigenous political agency has been undermined, leading to no clear road map for the future. The recent failure of the process to constitutionally recognise Indigenous peoples reflects deep institutional resistance to recognising Indigenous rights in Australia. Political resurgence is required to challenge efforts to resist or create barriers to Indigenous aspirations.

In 'The serendipity of justice: the case of unaccompanied migrant children becoming "adult" in the UK', and drawing on work spanning a decade, Elaine Chase considers what 'practical justice' might mean for unaccompanied migrant young people becoming adult but with uncertain legal status in the UK. Presently, as they turn 18, young people may be forced to return to countries of origin or denied access to public resources. At this juncture the serendipity of justice comes to light, being arbitrated by multiple actors governing and/or connected to the different spheres of young people's lives. The chapter shows how chance and circumstance factors have implications not only for migrant young people but for notions of practical justice more generally.

In a chapter entitled 'Patient-reported measures as a justice project through the involvement of service-user researchers', Annie Madden, Paul Lennon, Cassie Hogan, Mel Getty, Max Hopwood, Joanne Neale and Carla Treloar report on work to develop new patient-reported measures of treatment experiences and outcomes among people who use alcohol and other drugs. Their chapter discusses why service users should be part of the research process when developing new patient-reported measures, what this can deliver, the tensions that might exist, and the lessons learned from using such an approach. Like several earlier chapters, it demonstrates how research is stronger when conducted in partnership with service users as part of a justice-based project.

The next chapter, 'Unequal justice: the effect of mass incarceration on children's educational outcomes in the USA', takes its starting point from the fact that in the USA, an African-American child is six times as likely as a white child to have an incarcerated parent. Parental imprisonment is a key contributor to racial differences in school achievement. Its author, Leila Morsy, makes a series of practical recommendations. These include:

repealing mandatory minimum sentences for minor drug offences and other non-violent crimes; dis-incentivising prosecutors to seek maximum penalties for drug crimes; and increasing funding to provide meaningful support to released offenders.

We conclude with two chapters that focus on major public health challenges. In the first of these chapters, Alex Broom, Assa Doron and Peter Aggleton examine antimicrobial resistance as a public health and social justice issue. Despite its growing significance and the impending global crisis around the proliferation of multi-resistant organisms in the developing world, rarely is antimicrobial resistance looked at through the lens of justice. Using India as a critical case study, 'Antimicrobial resistance, bacterial relations and social justice' examines the potential of antimicrobial resistance to reflect and reproduce both local and global disadvantage. The chapter documents key elements of the social justice model needed to tackle the issue.

The final chapter engages with the importance of optimism and hope in relation to practical justice concerns. Reflecting on three decades of work in sexual and reproductive health, Purnima Mane and Peter Aggleton document success in the face of adversity. Their chapter, 'Fostering change through the pursuit of practical justice in sexual and reproductive health and rights', argues that at a time when sexual and reproductive rights are being questioned, focusing on the positive changes achieved in the past can guide and inspire. The chapter uses examples from India and Mozambique to identify how approaching issues through a practical justice lens – and a commitment to sound evidence, good normative argument and the best mechanisms for achieving change – can accelerate success despite major difficulties.

In conclusion

When we first set out to develop this book, our goal was to provide insight into the different contexts in which the principles and practice of practical justice might contribute to social change. Quite deliberately, we aimed for diversity in the perspectives offered and the activities, programmes and interventions described – appreciative of the 'as yet to be finished' project of practical justice, and the differences of perspective (with respect to goals, strategies and outcomes) that have yet to be reconciled. We offer this volume, therefore, not as any definitive treatise or last word, but as a first step and stimulus for thought. If you feel inspired by the project that we and contributors outline, please join us and others who struggle to make the world a better place for all.

Part I

Perspectives and accounts

Chapter 1

Concepts of justice and practical injustices

Paul Patton and Jeremy Moss

The essays collected in this book address a wide variety of scenes of practical justice and injustice. Together they raise the question: what is meant by 'practical justice' and how does it relate to current philosophical approaches to justice? Is it, for example, a distinct object or sphere of concern about justice in the way that distributive, historical and relational or recognitive justice identify distinct approaches and different concerns about the requirements of justice? Or is practical justice better understood as referring to the issues that arise when we move beyond the simplifying assumptions of 'ideal' theory to consider the requirements of justice in the real world?

Before elaborating on these different ways to answer the question about what it is that is practical about practical justice, it will be helpful to consider further the most common approaches to justice in contemporary political philosophy: distributive justice, reparative justice and a third, more difficult to define, concept that involves adequate recognition of particular peoples or groups within a population. Whether we think of these as distinct concepts of justice or as distinct dimensions of justice, they raise different concerns about the requirements of justice even if, as we will suggest below, they are interrelated in various ways.

Distributive justice

Distributive justice concerns the division of the material and other benefits of living in organised societies. It is sometimes presented as involving the distribution of what are called primary social goods such as health, education, opportunities for employment and income, as well as the benefits and burdens of being a member of political society. Egalitarian theories of distributive justice such as that of John Rawls start from the presumption that society should be considered a fair system of cooperation among individuals, all of whom are of equal moral worth (Rawls 1999). No one person's life or project in life is worth more than that of anyone else. Many believe that no one should be disadvantaged through no fault of their own, a principle that provides a basis for policies designed to remove or to compensate for undeserved disadvantage, whether this is the result of poverty, disability or membership of a disadvantaged social group.[1]

When formulated with reference to citizens of a particular community, distributive justice also involves the formal rights and duties of citizenship, such as protection under the law, equal treatment before the law, the absence of explicit discrimination or unjustified differential treatment, as well as rights of participation in the political process. In the international sphere, given there is no global government to regulate how social goods are divided, there is considerable debate concerning how we ought to justify any allocation of resources. This is a particularly important debate given that so many of the disadvantages people suffer are the result of global forces such as trade, pollution and climate change. The types of justifications for global justice divide broadly into two (Sangiovanni 2007). On the one hand, there are relational justifications. Relationalists hold that the justification for the principles of distributive justice is determined by the types of practices that they regulate, which can be of three kinds. So, for instance, some relationists hold that there must be the right kind of shared social and political institutions that involve cooperation or reciprocity in order for distributive justice to apply. Others claim that duties of global justice are triggered when institutions have a 'pervasive impact' on the higher-order interests of others. Different again is the claim that the legitimate exercise of coercion is required to trigger duties of global justice. Much depends on what is meant by the 'right type' of shared institutions. Relational views also hold that the kinds of practices that exist between people might determine the value and type of certain sorts of goods that form part of the distributed outcome. Goods such as working conditions or relations with family might gain part of their value because of the importance and meaning that one culture places on them.

Non-relationalists, on the other hand, argue that it is not the relations that people find themselves in that matter, but that there are basic features of moral personhood that ground global distributive principles of equality. So, if everyone in the world shares 'morally relevant properties' (cognitive abilities, for example) and we ought to treat everyone as mattering to the same degree, we ought also to extend our distributive concerns globally (Caney 2005, p. 265). Non-relationalists sometimes appeal to the idea of the moral arbitrariness of being born in one country rather than another to ground claims of global distributive justice. In the same way that people in wealthy countries should not be denied equal access to goods because of their skin colour or location, the fact that one person was unlucky to be born into a desperately poor country with no resources and high mortality is simply morally arbitrary and should not determine the kind of life they have.

Historic injustice

Another dimension of justice emerges in the context of discussing past wrongs, whether against individuals, particular peoples or groups. The measures employed to address this kind of injustice, including forms of reparation, restitution or compensation, often rely on a principle of 'balanced reciprocity' that is found among the oldest recorded systems of justice (Johnston 2011). This is one of the most basic principles in civil law, underlying remedies for specific injuries or infringements of rights. The simplest case is restitution, which involves the return or replacement of a stolen item. The New Zealand political theorist Andrew Sharp suggests that reparation represents 'the pure form of conservative justice' that seeks to rectify past wrongs and to restore things to their rightful state (Sharp 1997, p. 37).

The restitution approach to historical injustice lies behind the common-sense view that, since colonisation involved the unjust appropriation of Aboriginal lands, a just settlement must begin with recognition of their historical claim to the lands and other goods that were stolen from them (Lyons 1977). The same principle has obvious application in those colonial situations where treaties were entered into and then not honoured. If, as is often the case, the lands that were stolen cannot simply be restored without further injustice to their present owners, the argument is that the past injustice can be addressed by way of compensation. While the past cannot be changed, the present can be altered so that it is as if the past injustice had not occurred.[2] Another approach to historic injustice stresses the connection to ongoing injustices and argues that not all acts of wrong-doing in the past merit reparation, but only those that contribute to inequalities of circumstance and opportunity that affect the lives of individuals in the present. This kind of argument, linking present inequalities to past injustice, provides the basis for claims to reparations for African-Americans, or global forms of compensation for colonised or dispossessed Indigenous peoples. On either of these approaches, historic injustice cannot be entirely divorced from distributive justice, since it presupposes the existence of prior rights or entitlements that were wrongfully infringed. It follows that reparative justice depends upon prior principles of just distribution. It is because such principles were not respected that there can be a case for wrongful infringement of rights.

Another contemporary instance of the application of a principle of historical injustice concerns the allocation of future greenhouse gas emissions rights in the context of avoiding dangerous climate change. Acknowledging historical injustice is often invoked as crucial in dividing the world's remaining carbon budget. The carbon budget represents the finite amount of greenhouse gases that humankind can emit, consistent with an acceptable likely rise in global temperatures.[3] For example, many claim that historically high-emitting countries should be allocated less of the remaining global carbon budget than historically low-emitting countries, who are often late industrialisers and/or former colonies. There are some well-known and powerful objections to using a principle of historical injustice in this context. Critics argue that the kind of responsibility for historical emissions that would be required to justify them is often limited or absent, for a number of reasons. For instance, high-emitting countries were 'excusably ignorant' of the effects of their emissions for much of the past. Also, many of the individuals and a significant number of the countries responsible for past emissions no longer exist. There are further reasons for thinking that, at least in some cases, the links between present countries and their high-emitting precursors are weak enough to preclude any responsibility of the former for the emissions of the latter. Nonetheless, historical responsibility remains an important principle because, while these objections have some force, their target has typically been historical emissions that occurred before 1990, when the Intergovernmental Panel on Climate Change released its first report, establishing a strong scientific consensus for the view that human-produced greenhouse gases were contributing problematically to harmful climate change. Of all of the carbon emitted by fossil fuel use and cement production since 1750, almost *half* has been emitted since 1990. In total, 415 gigatonnes (Gt) of carbon have been emitted since 1750 – over 200 GtC of that has been since 1990.[4] These kinds of considerations draw our attention to the scope of historical principles and questions concerning how they apply to different periods of history.

Relational justice

These points concerning excusable ignorance and past harms raise the question of whether we should confine our attention, and our limited resources, to dealing with present wrongs in the effort to bring about a more just future. In response to this kind of argument, one reason for being concerned about past injustices is that these have consequences that continue into the present. The case of historical carbon emissions shows that how we should act in the present is bound up with actions that occurred in the past. Another reason for being concerned about past actions is that the injustices themselves can and do continue. Later in this book, Darryl Cronin points out that rectifying past injustice in the Australian case not only requires addressing current disadvantage and forms of material inequality, but also requires 'recognition of political status and recognising Indigenous customs, heritage and property rights' (see Cronin, Chapter 11). This points to a further dimension that shows that the requirements of justice are not exhausted by equality of distribution or appropriate compensation for historical wrongs, namely recognition or recognitive justice.

In the case of colonised Indigenous peoples, for example, the concepts of distributive and reparative justice do not address the sense of injustice that flows from the belief that colonisation involved a violation of fundamental rights of Indigenous peoples, namely their right to live according to their own cultural values and their right to decide what changes, if any, to their traditional way of life should be effected in response to the European invasion. These are rights that European peoples have traditionally claimed for themselves. They were not accorded to the Indigenous peoples encountered by the British in Australia. In this sense, and in Australia, the relation between Indigenous peoples and the settler population always was and remains an asymmetric relationship between unequal parties.

At the heart of this unequal relationship is a failure of recognition. However, we need to ask what kind of recognition is at issue. The Canadian philosopher James Tully suggests that, among the many questions of justice that may be raised in relation to the situation of colonised Indigenous peoples, 'a certain priority is claimed for justice with respect to cultural recognition in comparison with the many other questions of justice that a constitution must address' (Tully 1995, p. 6). Tully argues that the question of justice for colonised Indigenous peoples is a special case of justice with respect to cultural recognition. To the extent that constitutional arrangements will determine the normative and institutional framework within which other questions of justice (with regard to the distribution of social goods and the rectification of historical justice) will be addressed, they are the primary determinants of just relationship between colonisers and colonised. To the extent that these arrangements are undertaken on the basis of a failure to recognise Indigenous culture, law and systems of government, the relationship with Indigenous nations is unjust.

However, recognition is a complicated process and its relationship to justice is not always straightforward. Just as the commitment to equality raises the further question famously articulated by Amartya Sen (1979), 'equality of what?', the commitment to proper recognition raises the question of who or what is to be recognised. As Cronin points out, in the case of countries established by colonisation, it is all too frequently only certain aspects of indigeneity and the history of Indigenous peoples that are to be recognised (Cronin, Chapter 11). Recent Australian governments have made it clear that constitutional and political recognition would only be acceptable to them so long as they were confined to symbolic acknowledgement of Indigenous peoples' prior occupation and relationship to country at the expense of more meaningful forms of recognition of sovereignty and rights to self-determination. The Canadian Aboriginal scholar Glen Coulthard criticises the politics of recognition on the grounds that it does not significantly modify the power relation established between coloniser and colonised (Coulthard 2014).

In another, not entirely unrelated, context, the question of who or what is recognised emerges in discussions of the poor, marginalised and otherwise damaged members of the social 'underclass' in Western societies. kylie valentine points out that even a theorist of justice as involving both distribution and recognition such as Nancy Fraser, turns out to be 'magisterially unconcerned with the everyday practices of the poor themselves' (see valentine, Chapter 6). How the behaviour and attitudes of the poor are understood is important for the understanding of the requirements of justice for them. There is an important dimension of practical recognitive justice that is played out in the form and operation of welfare policies, but also in the practices of advocacy and provision of welfare services, and in the kinds of training and guidebooks provided for human services and social workers (see Hugman, Chapter 8).

In the colonial case, too, there are connections between recognitive, historical and distributive justice. For Rawls, one of the primary social goods to which all citizens must have equal access is the social basis of self-respect, which includes the way in which basic social institutions deal with members of a particular cultural group. This aspect of distributive justice is closely related to cultural recognition and historical injustice. On the one hand, the conditions of self-respect are affected by the history of official treatment of a particular people or peoples. Timothy Waligore points out that the history of racist policies towards colonised peoples leaves a legacy that must be addressed if the conditions of self-respect are to be restored:

> Having once said that Native Americans were an inferior race who could not maintain themselves as independent societies or polities, and whose people should not be able to pursue their chosen way of life, the US has an obligation to repudiate this message. Affirmative steps need to be taken to repudiate the specific messages associated with the dehumanizing stigmas attached to Native Americans. Full inclusion against the wishes of Native Americans cannot be reasonably expected to provide the social bases of self-respect for them. This history means that adequate support for their self-respect would likely require, at minimum, self-government rights.
>
> (Waligore 2016, p. 57)

On the other hand, there is empirical evidence that the conditions of self-respect have a bearing on outcomes in relation to health and education.[5] Together, these connections provide a strong argument that better outcomes in relation to social indicators such as health, as well as adequate recognition, require stronger forms of Indigenous autonomy and self-government.

The locations of practical justice

One way to begin to answer the question about the nature of practical justice and its relation to substantive concepts of distributive, historical and recognitive justice would be to take up issues about the level of abstraction and scope of theories of justice. Rawls offers a version of the familiar hierarchy of levels or degrees of abstraction at which we can talk about justice in *Political Liberalism* (Rawls 2005), when he distinguishes between ideas, concepts and conceptions of justice. He explains that, along with the 'opinions' or 'settled convictions' of the more or less rational and reasonable individuals who live together in political societies, ideas of justice provide the raw material that philosophy works up into successively more specific 'concepts' and 'conceptions' of justice. By 'ideas' he means relatively indeterminate and often fundamental objects of belief and value, such as the idea that justice is a matter of giving everyone their due, the idea of society as a fair system of cooperation over time, or the idea of citizens as free and equal persons. 'Concepts' then specify the meaning of the general terms employed in elaborating such ideas in particular contexts. For example, the concept of justice as applied to social institutions means the absence of 'arbitrary distinctions between persons in assigning basic rights and duties' and the existence of mechanisms for achieving 'a proper balance between competing claims'. Finally, 'conceptions' include, in addition to such meanings, particular principles and criteria for deciding 'which distinctions are arbitrary and when a balance between competing claims is proper' (Rawls 2005, p. 14 fn).

In these terms, Rawls's theory of justice as fairness spelt out in terms of his liberty and difference principles is a conception of distributive justice. We can imagine the same kind of differentiation of levels of abstraction in relation to historical and recognitive justice. Waldron's discussion of rational choice approaches to the problem of restoring the present to the way it might have been if particular historical injustices had not occurred, is an attempt to move beyond the concept of restitution towards a more developed conception of historical justice (see note 2). Tully's principles of recognition, consent and continuity as the basis for a just relationship between colonial and colonised peoples amount to elements of a conception of recognitive justice in the colonial context.

In each case, too, we can raise questions about the practical application of the principles that spell out a given conception of distributive, historical or recognitive justice: how are these to be applied in a given context and by what mechanisms is justice to be achieved? As a number of the chapters in this book demonstrate, efforts to achieve justice can all too often exacerbate problems or generate other injustices. For example, Thomas and Hansford in Chapter 4 point to ways in which efforts to achieve justice or parity in the treatment of mental and physical illness can lead to the pathologisation of stress on individuals, thereby diverting attention from distributive injustices that produce those forms of stress.

It follows that practical justice should not be considered another kind of justice alongside the distinct objects of distributive, historical and recognitive justice, but rather a complex level or field of determination that arises after the specification of any particular conception of justice. In more colloquial terms, we might suggest that practical justice refers to the point at which abstract principles meet social realities, or that justice becomes practical when the rubber that encases the wheels of government policy meets the social road.

A further feature of Rawls's approach that is relevant to this way of locating practical justice is the idea that the primary subject of justice is the institutional structure of society, where this includes not only the formal institutions of government but the social policies enacted through them. In these terms, we can say that principles of justice refer to the institutions and policies that a given conception of justice tells us would be required for a just society, while practical justice refers to the variety of issues that arise in the actual operation of those institutions and policies, including their application to particular problems, conflicts, populations and individuals.

One of the criticisms of Rawls's conception of justice put forward by Amartya Sen relates to its strong focus on institutions at the expense of consideration of the actual behaviour of individuals and groups in society. By taking the 'basic structure of society' as the primary object of a theory of justice, this conception leaves aside questions about the actual behaviour of agents involved in those institutions. Maffetone summarises this criticism by suggesting that 'Sen's main disagreement with Rawls lies in the thesis that fairness should also properly apply to persons whereas Rawls' principles apply only to institutions' (Maffetone 2011, p. 123).

Whether or not this is a justified criticism of Rawls, it does point to a distinctive field of practical justice issues that involves the *sociology of institutions* and how they *operate*. Elaine Chase's discussion of the situation of unaccompanied immigrant children raises questions about the social processes that in practice mediate people's access to rights that are supposed to ensure just treatment. She draws attention to the difference between the rights of individuals as enshrined in law, the 'rights' that moral theory and widely shared beliefs might assign to individuals, and the conditions under which legal and moral rights are made available, or not, to relevant individuals. She points out that the degree to which and the manner in which child migrants are able to take advantage of formal rights is

> ... stratified in an infinite number of other complex and dynamic ways from the moment they enter the country. In order to exercise rights as potential refugees, young people require the assistance of lawyers

who believe them; interpreters who do justice to their accounts of what happened to them; immigration officials who are empathetic and allow them to speak about what has happened; and sometimes medical specialists who will attest to them being the age they claim to be or confirm the extent of the trauma they have endured. Hence, in order to exercise their rights as children, young people in the first instance need to be believed by immigration officials and social services employees.

(See Chase, Chapter 12)

Once accepted as residents, children need access to a range of other service providers to ensure their equality of access to primary social goods such as health, education and income. The broader issue here is that of the social, political, institutional and interpersonal circumstances under which formal, legislated rights are accessible by individuals. The case of child migrants shows that their access to justice depends not only on social service departments of local authorities that are adequately resourced, but also on 'social workers who are compassionate towards them and who prioritise their needs, rather than those of the institution', not to mention a range of legal officials and civil society organisations and staff who can intervene to protect their rights and entitlements when necessary (see Chase, Chapter 12).

Another significant field of practical justice involves *policy choices* on the part of governments which affect the way in which institutions operate. So, for example, Ilan Katz (Chapter 9) points out that while it is widely accepted that governments should protect children against harm, a variety of different strategies have been adopted to achieve this goal. One approach treats child protection on the model of rescue or police operations, where the focus is on the discovery of harms, the identification of those responsible, and the determination of appropriate remedial operations. Another approach treats child protection on the model of public health, where the focus is on the discovery of risks and identification of ways to minimise these before harm occurs. As Katz shows, both strategies have strengths and weaknesses, and recent child protection policies have sought to mobilise elements of both, depending on the kinds of harm addressed. Both strategies also give rise to conflicts with other considerations of justice, including the rights of families, the rights of child protection workers and those of the broader community that bears the costs both of child protection and the failures of child protection.

These conflicts are in some ways analogous to the difficulties encountered by Rawls in his efforts to accommodate the feminist criticism of Susan Moller Okin (1987, 1989) and others that his theory of justice as fairness did not adequately address the inequalities produced by the gender system in modern European-derived societies. In part, the problem

turns on the ambiguous status of the family in relation to the basic structure of society. In his posthumously published lectures, *Justice as Fairness*,
Rawls explicitly includes the family in the basic structure of society on the
grounds that one of its important functions is to ensure the reproduction
of society and culture through providing for the upbringing of children
and ensuring their moral development and education. The family 'plays a
key role in the inculcation of a sense of justice and the political virtues
that support just political and social institutions' (Rawls 2001, p. 163).
Since it is part of the basic structure of society, it follows that the family is
subject to the principles of justice.

At the same time, he argues that, as in the case of many associations
such as the army, police forces or universities, these principles should not
apply directly to the internal life of the family. Rather, the political principles of justice are supposed to 'impose essential constraints' and
'guarantee the basic rights and liberties and fair opportunities of its
members' (Rawls 2001, p. 164). Husbands and wives are equally citizens
and the internal operation of family life cannot violate the basic rights of
either party. Since the aim of modern 'property-owning democracy' is full
equality of women, they should not be economically disadvantaged by
family arrangements which enable fathers to leave with their earning
power and accumulated assets. However, Rawls argues that the question of
how best to achieve such economic equality between husbands and wives
is 'not for political philosophy to decide' (Rawls 2001, p. 167). Similarly,
he argues that children must be subject to certain protections, but it is not
for political principles to regulate how parents treat their children: 'at
some point society has to trust to the natural affection and goodwill of
parents' (Rawls 2001, p. 165). At this point, we face a choice between considering practical justice as a further level in philosophical thought about
justice and, as Rawls sometimes appears to suggest, the limits of philosophical inquiry into the nature and principles of justice. At the very least,
he appears to leave room for a practice of justice that is informed by political philosophical principles but not determined by them.

The conflicting demands of justice in relation to child protection
arise even in the ideal case of culturally homogeneous communities
where there is widespread agreement over the rights of families and the
best interests of children. They are magnified and further complicated
in the case of *non-ideal societies* with *multicultural populations* where there
is often over-representation of children of minority ethnic and other
groups in child protection systems. In Australia, for example, there are
disproportionally more Indigenous children subject to child protection
than there are non-Indigenous children. At this point, the practice of
achieving justice in child protection becomes embroiled in the complexities of culturally diverse non-ideal societies, such as those established by
colonisation. Fundamental concepts such as the 'best interests of the

child', which is a basic concept embedded in the 1989 United Nations Convention on the Rights of the Child and has long served as 'a yardstick for guiding policy and practice in child care and protection', turn out to be contested concepts on which there is no cross-cultural consensus (see Katz, Chapter 9).

The complexity of real-world non-ideal societies poses significant challenges for citizens' access to primary social goods, particularly when we take into account the *broader social, economic and political contexts* that affect their availability. Health is both a human right and a primary social good, so there is no question that equal access to the basic conditions of health is a demand of justice in both domestic and international contexts. There is no justification for unequal access to conditions such as clean water, clean sanitation and conditions of life that allow for proper nutrition, adequate sleep, exercise and conditions of normal bodily and cognitive development. Equally, there is a *prima facie* right to medical services that seek to prevent as well as treat diseases. These are things that can and should be provided by governments in societies able to bear the cost of doing so. Of course, not all societies are capable of this, so inequalities in relation to the conditions of health arise between societies. Defenders of global justice claim that these should be addressed as matters of justice. However, there are many external conditions that contribute to such health-related inequalities in complex ways, including economic, social and political inequalities sometimes referred to as 'pathologies of power' (Farmer 2004). These pathologies also interact with and contribute to inequalities in other areas that affect the basic conditions of life for individuals and populations, such as the differential impact of climate change, environmental damage and pollution on national populations. An even more specific problem discussed by Broom, Doron and Aggleton is the differential development of antimicrobial resistance and its consequences for the unequal health of populations around the world. What is required, they argue, 'is an approach that brings together broad-ranging and community-specific data concerning the (social and biophysical) manifestations of antibiotic resistance and its effects with considered attention to what *should* be done in the context of global inequality' (see Broom *et al.*, Chapter 15).

Practices required to give effect to acknowledged rights

The existence and nature of human rights is now well established in international law and the practice of governments, although by no means universal. Human rights documents have provided both a foundation and a model for a number of declarations and conventions regarding rights of particular categories of persons, such as the Convention on the Rights of the Child (1989), the Convention on the Rights of Persons with Disabilities

(2006) and the Declaration on the Rights of Indigenous Peoples (2007). They have also provided a basis for international conventions against Genocide (1948), Torture (1984), Transnational Organized Crime (2000) and Corruption (2003). In all cases, questions arise about the mechanisms, means and practices required to give effect to such instruments and ensure in practice the equal rights of all persons. In relation to some internationally acknowledged rights, such as the rights of Indigenous peoples, the measures required to give effect to them include giving recognition and voice to the peoples concerned in the practices and policies of governments that concern them, in effect a form of practical recognitive justice. In relation to other internationally acknowledged rights, measures required to give effect to them involve changing the attitudes of those engaged in administrative, policing or other functions of governments.

Consider the human right not to be tortured, widely regarded as one of the most well-established principles of international law, public political reason and justice. The practice of torture has been prohibited by law and by international agreements such as the United Nations Convention against Torture (1984). The practical justice concern, in both domestic and international contexts, is how one goes about giving effect to this right. Celermajer points to the range of factors that may contribute to enabling the practice of torture in a given context, including such things as

> political interference in the work of law enforcement agencies; clientism and cronyism, whereby local political leaders used the police to prosecute their partisan interests; social norms concerning righteous violence against so-called delinquent individuals such as drug addicts; the admission by courts of evidence obtained under torture; the unwillingness of allied professionals such as doctors to document torture when they suspect it as having occurred; the fact that local police stations need to meet quotas of charges laid if they are to receive resources; intra-organisational violence; boredom and isolation of security sector personnel; and the lack of investigative skills amongst frontline police personnel.
>
> (Celermajer, Chapter 5)

Celermajer advocates an ecological or systemic understanding of the ways in which such arrays of enabling conditions surround and influence the behaviour of individuals. Only interventions in particular contexts informed by such systemic understanding can hope to change the behaviours involved in the practice of torture. It is at this level – well below the moral and other arguments deployed by philosophers to justify the existence of human rights, and below the 'macro-analysis' of societies and institutions at which theoretical criticism of human rights approaches to injustice are deployed – that it is possible to talk about effective practices of torture prevention.

These discussions raise an important issue concerning how basic principles of distributive justice can act as both a guide to how societies ought to organise rights and resources, and a reflection of the key concerns that different groups in society hold. An example of this tension concerns the kind of goods in terms of which individuals ought to be equal. An influential way of formulating such a list that contrasts with Rawls's method is the capability approach developed by Amartya Sen. Very briefly, in discussions of wellbeing, equality and development, and in many settings of practical justice, capabilities have been advanced as a way of capturing important dimensions of human ends while preserving the diversity of those ends. In the article that originally articulated the approach, Sen engaged in reflection on some of the alternative ways of conceiving equality while also setting out the elements of the metric (Sen 1979). The capability approach that he develops in that paper tries to steer a middle course between the other metrics that are typically put forward as an answer to the 'equality of what?' question – resourcism (for instance, Rawls's 'primary goods' approach) and welfarism (the view that equality ought to be seen as a matter of satisfying either preferences or subjective mental states) (Rawls 1999).[6] His well-known response to the question 'equality of what?' concentrates on what goods or states of affairs *do* for a person, rather than on the person's welfare or bundles of primary goods.[7] As Sen (1993, p. 30) puts it, '[t]he capability approach to a person's advantage is concerned with evaluating it in terms of his or her actual ability to achieve various valuable functionings as a part of living'. Equality of capability entails that individuals have equal freedom to achieve relevant 'beings' and 'doings'.

Yet, as influential as the capability approach continues to be, there remains a question about how we can select an appropriate list of capabilities from among the vast array of potential capabilities. Here, very simply, is the problem. There are two methods for selecting a list of capabilities and each takes us in a different direction. There is the subjective approach, sometimes endorsed by Sen, where it matters that the list of capabilities is subjectively endorsed and selected by individuals (Sen 2009). This approach argues that what is on the list is a matter for people to decide for themselves. There is also the objective approach endorsed by Martha Nussbaum (2011) and Elizabeth Anderson (2010), which claims that there is an objective list of capabilities that is independent of people's choices. Nussbaum's list is Aristotelian in the sense that it is a product of what she conceives of as being truly human. Anderson's method for selecting a list is closely tied to the objective interests we need to function as equals in a modern democracy.

We might understand this problem in terms of the employment of two distinct but related concepts: namely, *justification* and *legitimacy*. The philosopher A. J. Simmons has argued in another context that we need to distinguish between the justification of states, which is generic and refers to the benefits they provide for those subject to them, and the legitimacy of states, which is transactional and refers to the relationship between an individual and a given state (Simmons 1999). Here, Simmons is discussing the state and not equality, but we can also see that his distinction nicely captures a problem that faces many theorists of practical justice. On the one hand they want the elements on the list of equality to actually be good for people and morally permissible (Justified), but they also want them to be legitimate in the sense of having an appropriate level of endorsement. In these terms, we can say that people should have a say about important factors that have an impact on their lives. Legitimacy identifies something fundamental and desirable in a democracy because it focuses on an important aspect of the moral relationship between a state and its subjects. In many practical contexts in which justice matters, theorists and practitioners are faced with just this type of dilemma.

Conclusion

The move from fundamental ideas such as a belief in equality or society organised in a fair way to more concrete concepts and conceptions is a vital one for our understanding and practice of justice. What many of the issues discussed in the chapters in this collection demonstrate is a strong commitment to just outcomes in specific areas. In doing so they often rely on fundamental ideas, such as equal treatment or respect for diversity. Taking the steps from these general ideas to formulating them into a conception that balances different demands of justice is already a complex and difficult process, as the debates in political philosophy post-Rawls have shown. Taking the further steps required to give effect to principles of justice in actual societies rather than the ideal models of society relied on by political philosophers introduces new dimensions of complexity. Non-ideal societies have complicated histories that result in multicultural populations, diverse relations to other societies and to increasingly interlinked economic, political and environmental systems. These give rise to new forms of interaction between existing injustices, and new kinds of injustice, that create new problems in attempting to balance practical concerns with the demands of competing concepts. Being 'practical' about justice requires that we have an understanding of the conditions that generate these problems, of the constraints imposed on our responses by the demands of using concepts consistently, and of the forms of feedback produced by particular policy responses to injustice that give rise to what are often called 'wicked' problems. Together, these requirements challenge the idea that ideal theories provide us with the resources needed to achieve just outcomes in non-ideal societies. They force us to consider whether practical justice is the kind of thing about which there could be a theory, or whether we should think of practical justice as an open-ended assortment of policies, practices and practical maxims intended to address particular injustices in particular contexts. Either way, practical justice is a topic that calls for more investigation, both practical as well as theoretical.

Notes

1 Many also believe that we should extend concern to some disadvantages that are caused by an agent's choices, as choices themselves can be caused by factors outside an agent's control. See Moss (2014, ch. 3).
2 Jeremy Waldron attributes this approach to Robert Nozick, before going on to point out difficulties with the kind of counter-factual reasoning required to make the present accord with a different past (Waldron 1992, pp. 7–14).
3 We adopt the 2°C target here in line with the United Nations Framework Convention on Climate Change (UNFCCC) Paris Agreement negotiated in 2015.
4 Boden *et al.* (2016).
5 'When Native nations make their own decisions about what development approaches to take, they consistently out-perform external decision makers on matters as diverse as governmental form, natural resource management, economic development, health care, and social service provision' (The Harvard Project on American Indian Economic Development, About Us, Overview.
6 For a discussion of the concept of welfarism, see Sumner (1996).
7 For a list of some applications of the approach, see United Nations Development Program (1990–2007).

References

Anderson, E., 2010. Justifying the Capabilities Approach to Justice. In: H. Brighouse and I. Robeyns, eds, *Measuring Justice: Primary Goods and Capabilities*. Cambridge: Cambridge University Press, 81–100.
Boden, T. A., Marland G. and Andres, R. J., 2016. *Global, Regional, and National Fossil-Fuel CO₂ Emissions*. Oak Ridge, TN: Carbon Dioxide Information Analysis Center, Oak Ridge National Laboratory, U.S. Department of Energy.
Caney, S., 2005. *Justice Beyond Borders: A Global Political Theory*. Oxford: Oxford University Press.
Coulthard, G. S., 2014. *Red Skin White Masks: Rejecting the Colonial Politics of Recognition*. Minneapolis, MN: University of Minnesota Press.
Farmer, P., 2004. *Pathologies of Power: Health, Human Rights, and the New War on the Poor*. Berkeley and Los Angeles: University of California Press.
The Harvard Project on American Indian Economic Development. Available from: https://hpaied.org [Accessed 19 February 2019].
Johnston, D., 2011. *A Brief History of Justice*. Chichester: Wiley Blackwell.
Lyons, D., 1977. The New Indian Land Claims and Original Rights to Land. *Social Theory and Practice*, 4 (3), 249–272. Reprinted in J. Paul, ed., 1982. *Reading Nozick: Essays on Anarchy, State and Utopia*. Oxford: Blackwell.
Maffetone, S., 2011. Sen's Idea of Justice Versus Rawls' Theory of Justice. *Indian Journal of Human Development*, 5 (1), 119–132.

Moss, J., 2014. *Reassessing Egalitarianism*. Basingstoke: Palgrave Macmillan.

Nussbaum, M., 2011. *Creating Capabilities: The Human Development Approach*. Cambridge, MA: Harvard University Press.

Okin, S. M., 1987. Justice and Gender. *Philosophy and Public Affairs*, 16, 42–72.

Okin, S. M, 1989. *Justice, Gender and the Family*. New York: Basic Books.

Rawls, J., 1999. *A Theory of Justice, Revised Edition*. Cambridge, MA: Harvard University Press.

Rawls, J., 2001. *Justice as Fairness: A Restatement*. Cambridge, MA: Harvard University Press.

Rawls, J., 2005. *Political Liberalism: Expanded Edition*. New York: Columbia University Press.

Sangiovanni A., 2007. Global Justice, Reciprocity and the State. *Philosophy and Public Affairs*, 35 (1), 3–39.

Sen, A., 1979. Equality of What? In: I. S. M. McMurrin, ed., *The Tanner Lectures on Human Values*. Cambridge: Cambridge University Press, 194–220.

Sen, A., 1993. Capability and Well-being. In: M. Nussbaum and A. Sen, eds, *The Quality of Life*. Oxford: Clarendon Press, 30–53.

Sen, A., 2009. Capability and Well-being. In: A. Sen, *The Idea of Justice, Part III*. Harmondsworth: Penguin Books, 47–49.

Sharp, A., 1997. *Justice and the Māori: The Philosophy and Practice of Māori Claims in New Zealand since the 1970s*. 2nd edition. Auckland: Oxford University Press.

Simmons, A. J., 1999. Justification and Legitimacy. *Ethics*, 109 (4), 739–771.

Sumner, L. W., 1996. *Welfare, Happiness and Ethics*. Oxford: Clarendon Press.

Tully, J., 1995. *Strange Multiplicity: Constitutionalism in an Age of Diversity (1994 John Robert Seeley Lectures)*. Cambridge: Cambridge University Press.

United Nations Development Program, 1990–2007. *Human Development Reports*. Oxford: Oxford University Press.

Waldron, J., 1992. Superseding Historic Injustice. *Ethics*, 103 (1), 4–28.

Waligore, T., 2016. Rawls, Self-respect and Assurance: How Past Injustice Changes What Publicly Counts as Justice. *Philosophy, Politics & Economics*, 15 (1), 12–66.

Chapter 2

'Homeless women'

Histories of emotion and justice

Anne O'Brien

The November 2016 edition of the Australian current affairs magazine *The Monthly* carried an article entitled 'Rough Times'. Its subheading stated that homelessness had reached 'crisis levels' in the cities of Sydney and Melbourne. It was one of a genre: impelled by the desire to spread awareness of this searing problem, such articles usually focus on rough sleepers and almost always invoke a sense of crisis.

But while this rhetoric is not without political value, such writing is constructed on a contradiction that obscures deeper issues: for if we are in crisis mode, we have been so for a very long time. Homelessness in countries such as Australia did not become a problem between 2006 and 2011, as this article implied; nor in the early 1980s with deinstitutionalisation; nor indeed in 1974 when it was first legislated for by the Australian parliament. This is not to discount the role of neo-liberalism in shaping the current context, but to note that modern, industrial societies such as Australia have been living with this so-called 'crisis' for a long time, and it may be more productive to recognise that homelessness has become endemic. Such recognition does not discount the possibility of eradicating, or at least significantly reducing, the problem, but it does underline the fact that in order to do so – and to explain why that task has proven so difficult – it helps to deal in large scales of time.

This chapter seeks to contribute a depth of perspective to contemporary efforts to reduce homelessness by exploring the development of the term 'homeless' itself as a political label, focusing in particular on the emotions it evokes and their relationship with the pursuit of just outcomes. In this, it draws together fields that have rarely been treated together and have followed somewhat divergent affective paths. Since it appeared in the 1960s, labelling theory has mostly been used to explain how some groups become stigmatised as deviant, criminal or socially marginalised: the histories of clearly negative terms such as 'welfare dependency' and 'dole-bludger' are illuminating in this respect (Engels 2006, Archer 2009). Research on the history of emotions, however, has moved beyond concepts that openly stigmatise to examine the ambiguous effects of a range of feelings, including compassion and sympathy, though there has been little historical analysis of how emotions have shaped the shifting quest for practical justice (Rosenwein 2002, Frevert 2011).

The term 'homeless' is productive for exploring the connections between these fields because it is such a loaded and volatile term. A number of studies have discussed the significance of its contemporary uses, debating whether it is more or less likely to cast blame on people who are poor and considering what it means to those experiencing homelessness (Phelan *et al.* 1997, Walter *et al.* 2015). This chapter traces some of the ways a shift in its usage at the turn of the twentieth century panned out over the next 40 years, focusing in particular on how it affected women.

The word 'homeless' had long been used to refer to victims of war or natural disaster, but from the late nineteenth century it took off as a sociological descriptor. Unlike 'vagrant', it did not have a legal status and its implications were generally less pejorative. It was used by Charles Booth (1889–1903) in his 1890s social surveys of London, in contrast to Mayhew's (1985 [1849–50]) preference for 'vagrant' 40 years earlier, and it formed a chapter title in Salvationist William Booth's *In Darkest England* (1890). Over the next decades, 'homeless' became more widely used in transatlantic sociologies: Alice Willard Solenberger's *One Thousand Homeless Men* (1911) was one of the first texts to make 'the homeless' a discrete subject of study, and the Chicago sociologist Nels Anderson's *The Hobo: The Sociology of the Homeless Man* (1923) became a classic.

Emotion figures strongly in this shift. As Ute Frevert (2011, pp. 181–185) has argued, the growing momentum of compassion, and its near relatives sympathy and pity, began in the movement to abolish slavery and came to permeate the vast outpouring of nineteenth-century philanthropy. And yet racism and theories of hereditary deficiency were also products of the late nineteenth century, conduits for emotions such as anxiety and contempt. They too shaped this field, working to sustain the older category 'vagrant' as a figure of fear and indignation, not just among political conservatives, but among British Fabians and the working-class press (Vorspan 1977). Indeed, as 'the homeless' became more deserving in the first decades of the twentieth century, it would seem that 'the vagrant' became less so. This divergence is clear from the recommendations of the watershed report of the British Royal Commission on the Poor Laws and Relief of Distress 1905–09: with its specification of old age pensions for the worthy and labour colonies for 'the good-for-nothing loafer'. In settler colonial Australia, the rolling impacts of modernity, respectability and racism led to tighter public order laws and new Aboriginal 'Protection' laws to control Indigenous and settler 'vagrants' (Garton 1991, Broome 2010). The context in which homelessness was understood, then, was loaded, mercurial and contingent, but shaped by hardening lines of political categorisation.

These understandings were complicated in the case of women by the deep ideological conviction that they were naturally connected to home – simultaneously its guardians and in need of its protection. Reaching its height in the mid-nineteenth century, this belief made the position of 'the woman outside' particularly invidious (Golden 1992). And yet by the end of the century, reforms to women's legal and educational status and the backlash they generated, shifted the context in which such women were understood. In broad terms, the 'woman vagrant' remained liable to contempt, while the 'homeless woman' was more a figure of pity. But systematic searching of newspapers, facilitated by the Australian National Library's electronic index *Trove*, suggests that the 'homeless woman' was a flexible figure, whose emotional resonances were deployed by different interest groups for different political ends. Like 'the woman vagrant', she aroused anxiety but for her there was more hope and in some contexts she demanded justice.

Pity and anxiety: 'homeless women' considered

A small swag of reflective articles, most of which appeared in the *Sydney Morning Herald (SMH)* in the Federation decade (1900–10), provide a useful starting point for understanding these complexities, for they used 'homeless' – in their titles or their text – to explore the threats to women's 'special relationship' with home. Indeed, they defined the 'homeless woman', not as deeply poor and without shelter, but as living apart from family. They clarify important aspects of the subject at a moment when the ideological context was highly charged.

One of the most fulsome articles, entitled 'Homeless Women', presented a précis of life in various sites – 'Board and Residence', 'Apartments' and 'Rooms to Let'. These were implied as being on an economic hierarchy but all their residents were described as having 'practically no homes in the truest meaning of the word' and as uniformly miserable. For the problems of this homeless woman were not financial, but emotional. Whether she had been out teaching, typing or sewing, there were no 'merry voices to greet' her at the end of the day, 'no soft little arms' to 'fling themselves about her neck'; rather she took her evening meal with 'uncongenial folk, too tired like herself to be entertaining', after which she retired to her room where she passed 'the rest of the lonely evening'. In contrast, the mother of a family may have been tired, sick of small economies and 'weary of thinking of new dishes from Monday morning to Saturday night', but she was 'fortunate'. She enjoyed 'the sweet comforts, the dear delights' of a home where she was 'curtained, shut in from the world', where she had a 'pretty garden' and where her family gathered around her table 'in merry mood' to 'chatter over the events of the day' (*Sydney Morning Herald*, 12 December 1906).

Another article, entitled 'Homeless Workers', conceded the attraction of the independent life – indeed with a trade or profession a woman could become 'joyfully independent'. The sting – and here it *was* economic – came in old age, for she would inevitably be displaced by 'the next generation', and if she had not established 'home connections' she faced 'the problem of destitution'. Indeed, the author of this article considered that the woman who failed in the effort to make herself independent had a 'much better outlook' than she who succeeded and 'outlived her usefulness' (*Sydney Morning Herald*, 18 September 1907). Another article broached the difficulties facing a woman who sought to establish her own home. Here, financial difficulties receded again but emotional problems loomed large. Not only was public opinion against her, but she knew 'in her heart of hearts' that her 'nest' would 'never be just the same as the one built by two'. She was 'brave' but also 'naïve' and a little eccentric, for 'the old world' had no interest in 'abnormal beings' who 'attempt[ed] to violate' convention. The article reached a happy conclusion, however, through its recourse to maternalist ideology: it was 'sometimes' possible for 'the lone woman's house to be a far truer home than the one built by two' if it was a place where her 'mother instinct – which is a part of all real women' – could make it into a 'place of peace' where she took 'the waifs of life' and other 'homeless ones' under her wing (*Sydney Morning Herald*, 22 April 1908).

These articles were part of an ongoing discussion about the place of the single woman in *fin de siècle* Australia, stimulated by the disruptions of feminist activism (Magarey 2001). From the late nineteenth century onwards, major reforms admitted women to university, allowed them to control property and to sue for divorce on the grounds of cruelty or desertion, and in Australia women were among the earliest internationally admitted to the franchise in 1902 (Lake 1999). But these reforms were not won without struggle and various forms of backlash ensued. In a context of depression and economic rationalism, married women were purged from the New South Wales public service in the 1890s, and in a landmark case in 1907 the arbitration court defined a family wage as necessary for a man to support his wife and two children, signalling the institutionalisation of women's wage dependence over the next half century (Deacon 1989). In all this, Australia's geo-political context lifted the stakes and sharpened the tensions, its proximity to Asia and its declining birth-rate reinforcing the dedication to domestic ideology (Lake and Reynolds 2008).

The *SMH*'s reflections on the 'homeless woman' can best be understood in this context. As Katie Holmes has argued, a 'set of words' was commonly used to describe single women: marginal, peripheral, old maids, rejected, surplus, extra, superfluous, on the shelf, redundant – all signifying her personal and national marginality (Holmes 1998, p. 75). 'Homeless' is not on this list, and indeed it was not frequently used in this context. But its use at all was significant: indeed, likening her to the woman without shelter suggests that while her enemies may have wished to marginalise her, the single woman was in fact a disturbing presence. Calling her 'homeless' was a telling choice.

Brief newspaper reports of women without shelter over this period provide insight into what this connection implied. These women were almost always figures of pity. Many were ill, some were suffering from exposure, quite a few were found unconscious, some had died. In keeping with T. W. Laqueur's (1989, p. 204) theory that the details of bodily pain elicit 'sympathetic passions', the reports frequently described their physical state: 'careworn and emaciated' (*Argus*, 11 October 1913); 'deaf and dumb' (*Queensland Times*, 6 April 1926); 'lost her memory' (*Border Morning Mail and Riverine Times*, 12 July 1912). Women were frequently represented as victims of institutional indifference: badly treated by a hospital (*Ballarat Star*, 18 January 1896); 'evicted' by City Council (*Tamworth Daily Observer*, 8 September 1911); or refused refuge by charity: 'Shame on Salvationists' declared the populist *Truth* (25 December 1904). They could be victims of fate: 'motherless and homeless' (*Queensland Times*, 16 July 1913); or of heartless in-laws (*Telegraph*, 20 May 1902). Some were victims of fire (*Worker*, 29 August 1907); some of murder (*Singleton Argus*, 10 May 1929); some of desertion (*Daily Telegraph*, 24 July 1912). It was not uncommon for them to approach the police for help.

Such images haunted the *SMH* articles. In them, 'homeless' acted to scandalise but also to warn. And like these short reports, they depicted their subjects as figures of pity. Indeed, compared with many more openly disparaging articles, these were sympathetic to the problems facing single women. But while they all used pity, they did not use it in the same ways. The woman in the anti-lodgings article was unequivocally a figure of pity for she was 'compelled to be homeless' from 'one cause and another' (*SMH*, 12 December 1906). Like the women without shelter, she was the victim of forces outside her control. In the other articles, however, the women were given some choice and the authors presented them with options: the woman facing penury in old age was advised to 'more strenuously qualify' herself so that she could accumulate enough for retirement; the woman householder was advised to make her home a community, with herself as the maternal figure at its centre. Both solutions required the woman to change without contemplating any modification to the social order. And neither offered hope to women without financial resources. Their overriding message was that the independent route would have dubious outcomes, not only for herself but also for the wider society. Thwarting the 'mother instinct' threatened the quality of the social fabric and led to the decline in the birth-rate. In this context, then, pity worked to reinforce anxieties about the gender order and anxieties about 'an awakening Asia' (Pinto 2017, p. 108).

But if these articles can be read as 'sympathetic', a short piece in the *Newsletter* (12 March 1904), a nationalist paper founded by former *Bulletin* journalist John Haynes, was openly hostile. It used 'homeless' as an insult, to disparage women in the public sphere, declaring that 'the nice woman with the home-staying ways stops there', but 'meeting attending' women were the 'homeless camp follower[s] of society': lacking 'the great gifts of life – husband, children, a house to keep', they consoled themselves 'by adopting the world, its cares and sorrows'. Here pity was a tool of disdain, and 'homeless' encapsulated personal inadequacy: playing on the theme that women were chosen in marriage, she had been left on the shelf and her participation in public life was a pitiable compensation. And yet, while the tone of this article sets it apart from those in the *SMH*, they all closed off the independent woman's options in a shared context of social anxiety. If pity could idealise the subject, as Hoggett (2006, p. 154) argued, anxiety could urge it towards contempt. In all of these articles, pity was a sign of the distance between author and subject and worked to render the pursuit of justice irrelevant.

Justice and righteous anger: letters from 'homeless women'

In some ways the concerns of these articles resonate with contemporary understandings of homelessness: the boarding house is a recognised site of homelessness and the affective importance of 'home' is well established (Mallett 2004, Chamberlain and MacKenzie 2014, p. 78). But their sweeping generalisations obscure the range of historical experience. Seamus O'Hanlon's (2002) research on Melbourne in this period has shown that boarding houses covered a wide spectrum and at their higher end offered many satisfactions. Furthermore, while 'the family' could be a site of support it could also be a site of violence and oppression, as contemporary feminists well knew (Allen 1990, p. 44).

This is not to deny the inadequacy of low-end lodgings but to clarify what made them so. Central to housing deficiency was the domestic ideology encapsulated in the articles above. Entrenching the financially dependent wife as the norm, it provided justification for ignoring the acute shortage of housing for working women and wage levels insufficient for self-support. Women's wages were based on the assumption that they worked for 'pin money': one reformer described them as 'starvation wages' (Lockington 1917, p. 1). In fact, a 1928 study of women in the Victorian manufacturing industries found that 30 per cent of women were keeping, or helping to keep, family members (Cass 1983, p. 62). The pressure on housing came from the intersection of a range of conditions: accelerating urbanisation; the movement of women out of live-in domestic service and into factory work; and the statistical increase in the number of single women in the population – not just the women whose potential partners were killed in the war, but an earlier generation who reached adulthood in the 1890s and who were seen at the time as mounting a 'strike against marriage' (O'Brien 2017, pp. 4–5). But the government's preference for home ownership closed off the possibility of public support for alternative forms of accommodation. And dedication to domestic ideology ran deep, as seen in the decision made by the Australian Commonwealth Statistician not to count hotels and boarding houses as dwellings in the census as they did not 'represent the normal housing conditions associated with family life' (*Official Year Book* 1940, p. 561).

This was the context in which some women experiencing poor lodgings and low wages described themselves as 'homeless'. A batch of letters in the labour newspaper *Australian Worker* in 1918 provides rare insight into their world. That they appeared then probably reflects the increased unemployment and poverty produced by the war effort and the efforts of women trade unionists to get equal pay in the years before the war (Grimshaw *et al.* 1994, p. 210). Some of these letters were written by sympathetic wellwishers, but two were written by women experiencing these conditions. They, too, used 'homeless' to scandalise, but rather than warning against poor choices, they showed how limited the choices of working women were. They had none of the observers' detachment. They burned with a sense of injustice.

Their grievances extended from the nature of work to the prejudice they faced as single women. Declaring 'I am a homeless woman', 'Austral Maid' wrote of factories with 'hundreds of women herded together in a large, bleak, draughty room' with 'the endless whirr of machinery grinding out one's very soul' (13 June 1918). For 'Bell Bird', long hours working with machinery 'undoes the nerves' (20 June 1918). They gave no sign of pining for family life, but Bell Bird in particular resented the stigma attached to the unmarried woman: 'Nobody's woman! The hanger-on! The humiliated, hunted kind of being…' (2 May 1918). She resented 'friends of the masculine persuasion' on 'the Labour Platform' who 'refer to us as old maids' and who 'have been so busy making money that they have declared war on women' (2 May 1918). Austral Maid held 'capitalistic employers' to account and called on the 'smug comfortable other woman to help us break our chains' for it was 'slow murder, the way we live, and you who in safety allow this to go on, year after year, are all responsible' (13 June 1918). For these women, anxiety came not from gazing on suffering but from its hard experience. Both feared their capacity to sustain this working life into the future. Bell Bird worried that when her muscles 'wore out' she would be 'SCRAPPED' (2 May 1918).

In some senses these correspondents presented themselves as figures of pity, but they had a breadth of political perspective that focused on the structural conditions of injustice and their emotional outpouring was a collective plea on behalf of all working women. Bell Bird declared that women wanted 'the absolute return' for their work. She did not believe in 'tinpot reform, nor patchwork, nor tinkering' but thought that 'if we worked for use and not for profit, we should command houses of our own' (20 June 1918). Austral Maid also envisaged a holistic solution: she wanted to 'get the axe to the root by shortening the hours' and letting them 'share in the profits of their work makers!' Motivated by the desire for justice, their analyses went to the causes of women's homelessness: a domestic ideology that enshrined women's dependence and a gendered labour market.

Justice, compassion and shame: the 'homeless woman' out of work

In the depression of the 1930s, 'the homeless woman' reappeared in different form. Mass unemployment now meant that 'respectable' women – including those in lodgings – were forced to 'tramp the road', exposed to the risks of women without shelter. No longer confined to individual short press reports, the woman without shelter became a focus for the vulnerability of all working women. By 1933, female unemployment was 15 per cent – not including hidden employment – and emergency shelter was in high demand (*Census*, 1933, p. 1776). Organisations ranging from churches to political parties made efforts to provide hostel accommodation, as did individual advocates in local communities (O'Brien 2017, p. 9). They had varying degrees of success, but two of the hardest working advocates, Barbara Grahame in Newcastle and Marion Steel in Brisbane, illuminate the context of the quest.

Both communicated a sense of urgency and both were impelled by a sense of injustice: it was blatantly unfair that there were shelters for men but not for women. They elaborated individual cases of bodily suffering, telling, for example, of a tramping woman whose 'stockings were in shreds … and glued to her feet with blood' and sometimes calling on specific individuals to help (*Newcastle Morning Herald*, 27 May 1933, 20 February 1935). They both saw the sheltering of homeless women as a community responsibility but, reflecting Newcastle's radical tradition, Grahame was more critical of the broader social order and her language was stronger. She denounced 'this savage system that starves, brutalises and prostitutes' and made effective use of the vernacular: we 'are not even a Christian's boot lace' if we ignore poverty (*Newcastle Morning Herald*, 27 May 1933, 26 February 1935).

As in many of the voluntary initiatives that emerged in the depression in the face of limited government action, the helpers were struggling themselves. Grahame and Steel both admitted to having 'financial difficulties': Grahame's life was described by one of her admirers as 'extraordinarily hard' (*Newcastle Morning Herald*, 17 July 1935). Steel was described by *Truth* in 1930 as 'on the verge of a breakdown in health' and the next year as 'absolutely broke' (7 September 1930, 7 May 1931). Indeed, they themselves became figures of sympathy, their vulnerability adding to their authority. Ever ready with a poignant phrase, *Truth* wrote of Steel as 'one slight figure who stands alone between these women and absolute destitution' and declared that 'she herself is as poor as any of them' (21 February 1932). Grahame drew on her own experience to reject the paralysis of pity: 'Don't just say "Oh poor thing" when hearing of a homeless girl. I've been "poor thinged" myself and it always rouses me to derisive scorn' (*Newcastle Morning Herald*, 26 February 1935).

Steel and Grahame were doubtless motivated by a sense of injustice but, unlike the correspondents to the *Australian Worker*, their vision was immediate and ameliorative rather than holistic and structural. Further, as advocates who sought to persuade the public to support these hostels, they relied on the support of local newspapers, which meant that in some ways they reinforced gender ideologies that opened the way to hiding and shame. Steel, for example, argued that homeless women wanted to keep their situation hidden. 'Of course they do not desire any publicity', she wrote in 1930, 'in case it was considered a reflection on her character' (*Daily Standard*, 29 April 1930). MD, a correspondent in the Newcastle campaign, wrote that women 'shrank from voicing their sad plight through fear of what the conventional world thinks of a woman who tramps the road' (*Newcastle Morning Herald*, 9 April 1932). Another writer thought that homeless women 'hid their want from the majority of the community, particularly the men' (*Newcastle Morning Herald*, 10 April 1935). Steel was conscious of the distinctive problems of homeless women. They found it harder to approach strangers for help in the street because they would be thought immoral, and in cases when women were not ill enough for the invalid pension, nor old enough for the old age pension, 'their appearance is against them', they 'drift to hospital, prison or street' (*Daily Standard*, 28 August 1931). She thought that a woman was 'subject to many temptations when she is destitute and homeless' (*Telegraph*, 19 September 1935).

In making the case for shelter, then, these advocates trod a fine line between challenging and reinforcing the old nineteenth-century assumption that for women homelessness was a path to prostitution. They needed to draw the homeless woman to public attention while respecting her privacy and commending her discretion. Since it preserved the dignity of the individuals concerned, this sensitivity can hardly be deplored. But in the longer term it may have worked to reinforce shame and to sharpen the division between the respectable and unrespectable homeless woman. In this slippery context it is worth noting that advocates were acceptable as impecunious but they were not represented as 'homeless'.

Fear and contempt, fascination and pity: the 'woman vagrant'

All through this period, newspapers continued to publish short reports about the 'homeless woman'. But she had a negative counterpart in parallel short reports – the 'woman vagrant'. Both sets of reports were clearly labelled: those headed 'vagrant' generally carrying quite different emotional messages from those headed 'homeless'.

Most of the detail accompanying the woman vagrant cast her as a figure of fear and contempt rather than pity. She was likely to be described as 'dirty' rather than frail or emaciated: common tropes were 'drunken and filthy' and 'about the streets' (*Argus*, 7 October 1924). Some reports sought to shock – an old age pensioner was reported as hosting 'a drunken carnival' when she received her pension (*Mercury and Weekly Courier*, 13 December 1901). Some made jokes at the women's expense: magistrates' jibes were not uncommon. One case reported with some amusement over several weeks was of a 23-year-old who tried repeatedly to leave her 'hubby' and kept being found without means of support by police (*Daily Standard*, 22 July 1930). Some were more voyeuristic than others. 'Girl vagrants' were always good copy, particularly if they were suspected of having sex with foreigners. Cases of inter-racial marriage also got space. Elsie Foo, described as 'a neatly dressed white woman' and 'a great friend of the Chinese', was arrested for drunkenness and having insufficient means of support in Bathurst in March 1925 (*Bathurst Times*, 11, 14 March 1925).

If the 'homeless woman's' desire to hide her shame became one of the markers of her deservedness, the woman vagrant could be seen as distinguished by the flagrancy of her public transgression. But the labels were not watertight and pity was not always absent. The woman vagrant who was disabled or mentally ill was sometimes referred to as 'unfortunate'. In some cases, pity worked to enhance fascination, as in the case of 'Bluey Ah Nat', a young Aboriginal-Chinese woman described in a series of articles as 'of diminutive stature', 'suffering from an incurable disease to her eyes' and not 'exactly right in the upper storey' (*Daily News*, 5 April 1897, 23 July 1897, 2 December 1899).[1] In others, it worked with disgust: one policeman reported watching while a woman picked up cigarette stumps in the street and smoked them and then drank methylated spirits – her hair was 'matted' and she had 'sores on her face' (*Evening News*, 17 January 1930). Those who fought back were less likely to evoke pity. In 1915, when a young girl with venereal disease who had just served a three-month sentence for vagrancy was ordered back to Pentridge for 12 months, 'she wept loudly and had to be escorted away', carried by two constables 'struggling, hitting, kicking and screaming all the way' (*Brunswick and Coburg Leader*, 24 September 1915).

In one sense the disdain directed towards the vagrant is not surprising, for vagrancy was a legal status. Indeed, the woman vagrant was frequently known to police, or found associating with people known to the police. One elderly woman had 60 convictions, and collectively the women were often described as 'old offenders' (*News*, 14 February 1925, *News*, 14 January 1929). Some behaviours were defined in the law, such as 'accosting men on the street', though sleeping out was more open to interpretation and it was not always clear why some were cast as vagrant (*Daily News*, 17 February 1931). Entrapped in the criminal justice system, the woman vagrant was excluded from visions of practical justice, whether ameliorative or structural.

Conclusion

If 'homeless' now seems a somewhat tired term of debatable value, it was relatively new at the turn of the twentieth century, at least in relation to deeply poor people in peacetime industrial societies. Reflecting a new chapter in the humanitarian narrative, it did not replace the older label 'vagrant' but came to be used alongside it. It had particular resonance for women. At moments of acute social anxiety, 'the homeless woman' commanded attention and sympathy. In the hands of the conservative press, however, she acted as a warning against female independence. To women associated with the trade union movement she was a rallying cry. To both, her continuous presence in short, distressing press reports threatened the descent imagined for all vulnerable women. Such fears seemed to materialise in the 1930s depression, when sufficient numbers of women were without shelter for their problems to penetrate public indifference and advocates emerged to prevent 'the homeless woman' from joining the ranks of 'the woman vagrant'. One of the great paradoxes in this story is that while a woman's place within a family was assumed to be her ultimate defence against homelessness, the economic conditions of family life were a major source of her precarity.

The cluster of emotions around 'the homeless woman' differed in each context and shaped advocates' stance on justice. In this their speaking position was crucial. To the detached observers in the *SMH*, the homeless woman was a subject of pity, not justice, but exploited women workers and depression advocates both sought just outcomes. Like those seeking practical justice today, their political stance was based on evidence and reasoned argument, but they were differently positioned and differently constrained. The voices from 'below' addressed structural inequalities but lacked the infrastructural support to disseminate their message; the depression advocates penetrated public discourse but had to tailor their message to be effective.

Contemporary advocates continue to debate the tensions between charity and justice in trying to eradicate homelessness (Parsell and Watts 2017). The case studies in this chapter shine a light on the role of gender in generating these tensions in the period before the post-war welfare state was established and before women's sexual liberation was on the feminist agenda. The 'big picture' provided by a historical perspective shows that those who experienced homelessness had the clearest vision of the inequities that lay at its core, suggesting that such voices ought not just to be heard, but called on to shape advocacy.

Note

1 This was one of the few references to an Indigenous woman under 'vagrancy'. Further research is needed into the relationship between the Protection Acts and the Vagrancy Acts and their reporting.

References

Allen, J., 1990. *Sex and Secrets: Crimes Involving Australian Women since 1880.* Melbourne: Oxford University Press.

Anderson, N., 1923. *The Hobo: A Sociology of the Homeless Man.* Chicago: Chicago University Press.

Archer, V., 2009. Dole Bludgers, Tax Payers and the New Right: Constructing Discourses of Welfare in 1970s Australia. *Labour History*, 96, 177–190.

Booth, C., 1889–1903. *Labour and Life of the People in London.* London: Macmillan.

Booth, W., 1890. *In Darkest England and the Way Out.* London: International Head-quarters of the Salvation Army.

Broome, R., 2010. *Aboriginal Australians: A History since 1788.* Sydney: Allen & Unwin.

Cass, B., 1983. Redistribution to Children and to Mothers. In: C. V. Baldock and B. Cass, eds, *Women, Social Welfare and the State in Australia.* Sydney: Allen & Unwin, 54–88.

Census of the Commonwealth of Australia, 1933, Part XXVI. Canberra: L. F. Johnston, Commonwealth Government Printer.

Chamberlain, C. and MacKenzie, D., 2014. Definition and Counting: Where to Now? In: C. Chamberlain, G. Johnson and C. Robinson, eds, *Homelessness in Australia: An Introduction.* Sydney: UNSW Press, 71–99.

Deacon, D., 1989. *Managing Gender: The State, the New Middle Class and Women Workers 1830–1930.* Melbourne: Oxford University Press.

Engels, B., 2006. Old Problem, New Label: Reconstructing the Problem of Welfare Dependency in Australian Social Policy Discourse. *Just Policy*, 41, September, 5–14.

Frevert, U., 2011. *Emotions in History: Lost and Found.* New York: Central European University Press.

Garton, S., 1991. Pursuing Incorrigible Rogues: Patterns of Policing in New South Wales 1870–1920. *Journal of the Royal Australian Historical Society*, 77 (3), 16–29.

Golden, S., 1992. *The Women Outside: Meanings and Myths of Homelessness.* Berkeley: University of California Press.

Grimshaw, P., Lake, M., McGrath, A. and Quartly, M., 1994. *Creating a Nation 1788–1990.* Melbourne: McPhee Gribble.

Hoggett, P., 2006. Pity, Compassion, Solidarity. In: S. Thompson, S. Clarke and P. Hoggett, eds, *Emotion, Politics and Society.* Basingstoke: Palgrave, 145–161.

Holmes, K., 1998. Spinsters Indispensable: Feminists, Single Women and the Critique of Marriage, 1890–1920. *Australian Historical Studies,* 29 (110), 68–90.

Lake, M., 1999. *Getting Equal: The History of Australian Feminism.* Sydney: Allen & Unwin.

Lake, M. and Reynolds, H., 2008. *Drawing the Global Colour Line.* Melbourne: Melbourne University Press.

Laqueur, T. W., 1989. Bodies, Details and the Humanitarian Narrative. In: L. Hunt, ed., *The New Cultural History.* Berkeley: University of California Press, 176–204.

Lockington, W., 1917. Starving Women and Starvation Wages. *Women's Social Work,* 2 (1), 1–2.

Magarey, S., 2001. *Passions of the First Wave Feminists.* Sydney: UNSW Press.

Mallett, S., 2004. Understanding Home: A Critical Review of the Literature. *The Sociological Review,* 52 (1), 62–89.

Mayhew, H., 1985 [1849–50]. *London Labour and the London Poor.* Harmondsworth: Penguin.

O'Brien, A., 2017. Homeless Women and the Problem of Visibility. *Women's History Review* (published online 26 October 2017 https://doi.org/10.1080/09612025.2 018.1392275).

Official Year Book of the Commonwealth of Australia 1940, 1940. Canberra: L. F. Johnston.

O'Hanlon, S., 2002. *Together Apart: Boarding House, Hostel and Flat Life in Pre-war Melbourne.* Melbourne: Australian Scholarly Publishing.

Parsell, C. and Watts, B., 2017. A Reflection on New Forms of Homelessness Provision in Australia. *European Journal of Homelessness,* 11 (2), 1–10.

Phelan, J., Link, B. G., Moore, R. E. and Stueve, A., 1997. The Stigma of Homelessness: The Impact of the Label Homeless on Attitudes towards Poor Persons. *Social Psychology Quarterly,* 60 (4), 323–337.

Pinto, S., 2017. The History of Emotions in Australia. *Australian Historical Studies,* 48 (1), 103–114.

Rosenwein, B. H., 2002. Worrying about Emotions in History. *American Historical Review,* 107 (3), 821–845.

Solenberger, A., 1911. *One Thousand Homeless Men: A Study of Original Records.* New York: Charities Publication Committee.

Vorspan, R., 1977. Vagrancy and the New Poor Law in Late-Victorian England. *The English Historical Review,* 92 (362), 59–81.

Walter, Z. C., Jetten, J., Parsell, C. and Dingle, G. A., 2015. The Impact of Self-Categorizing as 'Homeless' on Well-being and Service Use. *Analyses of Social Issues and Public Policy,* 15 (1), 333–356.

Chapter 3

Worlds apart and still no closer to justice

Recognition and redress in gendered disability violence

Leanne Dowse

Introduction

While it is widely recognised that violence and abuse are disproportionally experienced by women with disability (Commonwealth of Australia 2010), the specifics of this intersectional experience vary significantly among those affected. Drawing on a body of research addressing intersectional experiences of gendered disability violence, this chapter explores a troubling dichotomy in justice responses to disabled women that sees some excluded from processes of justice, while others are criminalised and intractably entrenched within the justice system. These contradictory trajectories are bound up in the deep and complex interconnections between disability, gender, social inequality and institutional ableism, the net result of which is pervasive systemic violence. Addressing the issue of gendered disability violence in all its guises requires careful interrogation of the ambivalence of frameworks and systems of justice in recognising and responding to diverse intersectionalities. I begin by sharing two stories of women with disability.

Lily

Following a radio interview to publicise a national symposium on gendered disability violence, I received an email from the mother of a woman with intellectual disability, which she gave me permission to share in an effort to bring issues of violence, gender and disability to light.

> My late husband and I set off on an around-Australia caravan trip and a social worker suggested our daughter would be well taken care of at [Disability] Department-run flats fairly close to our home as she did not want to travel and wanted to try and live more independently. What followed over the two years she was there has damaged her irreparably, both mentally and emotionally, and despite police statements about the sexual abuse, the Public Prosecutor rejected

proceeding against the carer/perpetrator on the basis that it was our daughter's word against his. The police were surprised as they absolutely believed her and could not understand why the case wasn't prosecuted. My daughter is very clear and knowledgeable about not only the sexual abuse but also the decisions made by those in control concerning every aspect of her life as well as the other disabled residents. We as a family feel utterly let down by the Justice system as well as the lack of accountability with regard to the staff in whose care we left our daughter.

Natalie[1]

Natalie's story has been compiled from a linked de-identified dataset bringing together extant administrative information from eight criminal justice and human service agencies about the institutional contacts for a cohort of individuals with known disability diagnoses who have been in prison in one Australian state. Natalie's story is therefore a partial account and does not include her own voice.

Natalie is a young woman with multiple cognitive and psychiatric diagnostic labels including intellectual disability, dissocial personality disorder, attention deficit disorder, emotionally unstable personality disorder, histrionic personality disorder and psychotic disorder due to the harmful use of cannabinoids. During her early years, Natalie attended a special class but due to 'abuse of staff' was repeatedly suspended and eventually excluded from school at the age of 14. From this time onwards, she was also unable to remain in the family home due to an aggravated relationship with her brother who had a mental illness. Her first contact with the police was at this time where she was identified as a victim of domestic violence and of sexual assault by her sibling.

During her teenage years Natalie had lengthy periods in out-of-home care and crisis accommodation where placements often break down due to aggressive behaviour. She was frequently identified as being homeless as a teenager. She had 22 contacts with Police before her first incarceration as a juvenile at 15, with seven episodes in youth custody over a four-month period at this time. During these periods, both in detention and in the community, there were multiple alerts and hospital admissions for self-harm and suicide attempts. During her residential placements, staff frequently called the police because of Natalie's damage to property and assaulting carers.

In her early adulthood Natalie experienced frequent domestic violence in her relationships and apprehended violence orders are also taken against her. She had three pregnancies, with all children being born by the time she was 23. Each of her children were removed. Natalie continued to have frequent police contact and to cycle in and out of custody as an adult.

That both Lily and Natalie experience forms of injustice in response to their experiences of gendered disability violence is clear; however, their experiences are worlds apart. While these differences are starkly connected to their social and personal positioning, what runs through both of their stories is the unsettling manifestation of the systemic ableism which sees violence against women with disability as in some way less important or less criminal than would be the case were it to be perpetrated against non-disabled women (Sherry 2000). Both stories highlight individual, institutional and systemic failures to practically recognise and address justice claims in relation to gendered disability violence.

Gendered disability violence

Gendered disability violence encompasses all forms of forceful, injurious or demeaning treatment towards disabled woman, which includes the full scope of violence as well as that which is gender-related or disability-related, and which occurs in the community and in domestic and institutional settings (Dowse *et al.* 2016). It is a phenomenon of compounded inequity arising from the cumulative impact of disability and gender discrimination (Price-Kelly and Attard 2010) and so requires intersectional analysis attuned to the ways in which oppressive institutions – including sexism and ableism – mutually construct one another (Meekosha and Dowse 1997). This prompts analysis beyond fixed identities that individuals 'have' or 'are' and draws attention to processes of entanglement (Lykkee 2010, p. 51), which extend to considerations beyond individual victim characteristics. These processes of entanglement can be seen in the stories of gendered disability violence experienced by Lily and Natalie, where the failures of just responses to their experiences are differentially distributed across domains of justice, including the structural, institutional and procedural.

The evidence

Women with disability have been identified as at significantly higher risk of violence and sexual abuse compared with their disabled male peers and non-disabled women (Commonwealth of Australia 2010), but its incidence remains largely under-reported (CRPD 2013). Although disabled women experience the same forms of violence as other women and girls, they also experience forms of violence that are particular to their situation of social disadvantage, cultural devaluation and increased dependency (Chenoweth

1997). Global studies suggest that women and girls with disability are twice as likely to experience domestic violence and other forms of gender-based and sexual violence as women without disabilities, are likely to experience violence over a longer period of time, and are likely to sustain more severe injuries as a result of the violence (Ortoleva and Lewis 2012).

Disabled women also experience violence that is specific to the nature of their disability. This can include, for example, denial of mobility and communication devices, the withholding of food or medication, threats of institutionalisation, threats to, and/or abuse of, support or assistive animals (WWDA 2011), restraint in order to administer non-prescribed medication, exploitation for financial gain (Dillon 2010), forced contraception, forced or coerced psychiatric intervention, medical exploitation, violations of privacy, humiliation and harassment (WWDA 2011). In addition to physical, mental and sexual violence and abuse, women with disability also face unnecessary institutionalisation, denial of control over their bodies, lack of financial control, denial of social contact, and restrictions on employment and community participation (INWWD 2013).

Much gendered disability violence is precipitated by the exposure of women with disability to care and support or control systems. Power differentials in institutional settings make those in health-related, disability-related, age-related, or criminal justice institutions more susceptible to violence, exploitation and abuse. Violence can be perpetrated with 'relative impunity' in institutional and care settings such as prisons and residential facilities, respite services, day centres, hospitals and special education classrooms that contribute to a perception of prisoners, patients and residents as powerless and exploitable people. Such facilities are largely populated by people who face significant disadvantage and vulnerability and who often experience poor health, physical and/or cognitive impairments, substance abuse issues, mental illness, low education, and who have faced myriad other disadvantages (Clark and Fileborn 2011). This vulnerability is further compounded by reliance on both informal and formal support and care within these settings.

In such spaces the involvement of the state and its institutions in this violence against disabled women is a central feature and is recognised by disability movements, who have fought long and hard for the closure of institutions (People with Disability Australia, n.d.), which numerous media reports and commissions of inquiry have demonstrated have frighteningly high levels of criminal assault, including sexual assault, and neglect associated with them. Legal and bureaucratic systems have been deeply implicated in some of the worst cases of violence, abuse and crimes, with sexual and physical assaults revealed to be a routine, sometimes daily, experience, and yet rarely addressed adequately by service staff or justice agencies. Sadly, this violence is often viewed as an administrative infringement to be dealt with as a managerial and personnel issue and is often not reported as a crime (Robinson 2013). When these actions are recognised as offences, those who commit them are often given lighter sentences than others who commit similar offences against non-disabled victims (Sherry 2000).

The criminal justice system is a space in which the connections between gender, disability, violence and social disadvantage are particularly evident. The majority of women in the Australian criminal justice system have been diagnosed with mental ill health and/or trauma, and the majority have a history of childhood violence and/or adult domestic violence (Stathopoulos 2012). As a space, the criminal justice system and specifically the prison have high concentrations of women with psychosocial disability who have experienced violence. Research on a cohort of imprisoned women with disability in the state of New South Wales in Australia (Dowse *et al.* 2015) indicates that the women with complex disability, social disadvantage and offending have an alarmingly high incidence of violent victimisation (79 per cent had at least one such instance) and that increasingly complex disability (having more than one diagnosis associated with intellectual disability, acquired brain injury or a mental health condition) is associated with higher rates of violent victimisation, whereby 76 per cent of those with one diagnosis, 87 per cent of those with two diagnoses and 92 per cent of those with three diagnoses had been victims of violence. High rates of violent victimisation were found to be particularly associated with being Indigenous, having ever been homeless, having been in custody as a young person, and having a diagnosed drug and alcohol issue.

Recognition and reporting of gendered disability violence

Women with disability often do not report the violence they experience as institutions of justice are not accessible (either physically or cognitively) and/or do not provide reasonable accommodation for women with different types of impairments (Ortoleva and Lewis 2012). Moreover, for many women these spaces do not provide a 'safe' space for the disclosure of their experiences. Disabled women also lack access to legal protection and representation, and law enforcement officials and the legal community are generally ill-equipped to recognise, understand and address issues of violence. The testimony of women and girls with disabilities may not be viewed as credible by the criminal justice system and lack of access to information in appropriate formats leaves disabled women marginalised within the system (Ortoleva and Lewis 2012). This in turn may heighten their risk of being seen by perpetrators as 'ideal victims' as they are either unable to report violence or not believed when they do so (Lund 2012).

This systemic incapacity to provide for just responses to gendered disability violence is underpinned by a lack of comprehensive prevalence data. For example, in Australia there is no nationally representative survey that comprehensively captures violence against women with disabilities. The Australian Bureau of Statistics does conduct the Personal Safety Survey (PSS), which collects data about the nature and extent of violence experienced by men and women from the age of 15. This records whether the respondent has a disability using standard activity restriction measures. However, the PSS has significant shortcomings in relation to gendered disability violence, including the fact that a large but unknown proportion of women with disabilities are under-represented because the survey (1) excludes those who need communication support to participate in a survey interview, (2) excludes people with a disability who usually reside in non-private dwellings such as institutions, and (3) only addresses experiences of physical violence and sexual violence and excludes from its measurement frame consideration of disability-specific violence, thereby excluding the very disabled women identified as most exposed to the risk of violence (Dowse *et al.* 2016). Public reporting of the PSS, by its relatively simplistic methodological approach, has been found to significantly under-estimate prevalence and incidence, where its aggregate reporting indicates 6 per cent prevalence of violence experienced by women with disability, while individual analysis reveals that 62 per cent of women with a disability under the age of 50 had experienced violence (Dowse *et al.* 2016, p. 350).

These frightening statistics and the human lives that sit behind them call for acknowledgement that prevailing conceptualisations, recognition and response to the needs and rights of women who have experienced or are at risk of experiencing gendered disability violence are clearly inadequate (Dowse *et al.* 2013). They point to the nature of such violence as pernicious, frequent and particularly complex, not least because its compounding fundamentals are embedded in normative systems of response which are deeply ableist, non-gendered and classist. This in turn gives rise to negative justice outcomes for disabled women such as Lily and Natalie, where their diverse intersectionalities lock them in to contradictory trajectories of exclusion and entrenchment.

Exclusion and entrenchment in the spaces of justice

Incomplete knowledge about gendered disability violence has led to its almost wholesale exclusion from the public policy arena, with significant consequences for effective recognition and response in spaces of justice. These axes of exclusion can be seen in the erasure of several critical dimensions of gendered disability violence, including its spatial dimension in non-domestic closed environments of care and containment, the narrow categorisation of violence which obscures specific forms of disability violence, and static understandings of the relational dimensions of violence whereby relationships of power, dependency and care are not considered in the identification of perpetrators. The key issue here, however, is not simply the 'grand erasure' of gendered disability violence, but more importantly the fact that the specificity of identities, socio-economic circumstances, spatial locations and relational contexts is simply not recognised. Where disability is present in relation to violence, it is considered incidental rather than constitutive. This is important because it is the intersection of gender and disability that is central in shaping the type, likelihood and incidence of violence for disabled women.

But this is not the end of the story for gendered disability violence, as we can see in the accounts of Lily and Natalie's experiences. While exclusion is writ large in Lily's experience, whereby her gender and disability intersect in ways that preclude her access to the positive processes of justice in the event of her experiences of violence, for Natalie, these identities are further entangled with social disadvantage and criminal offending. The outcome for Natalie is not simply exclusion from positive processes of justice, but rather, capture by and entrenchment in the justice system itself. Both Lily and Natalie experience these outcomes as further traumatising. For Lily this can be seen in her mother's observation that the experience 'has damaged her irreparably both mentally and emotionally', and for Natalie, observed in her lifelong self-harm, ongoing entanglement in offending and incarceration, and in state intervention via the removal of her children. Beyond individual trauma, these processes signal systematic, symbolic and institutional forms of violence that arise from the application of able-bodied un-gendered norms to the interrogation of gendered disability violence and to the remedies embodied in processes of justice.

Why do we need an inclusive justice-based approach?

As some disability theorists have begun to argue, traditional views of justice have often theorised people with disability as being beyond the scope of justice (Riddle 2014). Where scholars (e.g. Nussbaum 2011) have engaged with the issues, disability is dealt with as an exception, suggesting that the injustice of, for example, gendered disability violence does not bear a close resemblance to the forms of injustice experienced by able-bodied people. This failure of inclusion in theories and practices of justice has the default consequence of shifting the focus on the causes of injustice to individual deficiencies (Lily not being a reliable witness to her violence) or to holding people individually responsible for their poor choices (Natalie's use of drugs or her choice of relationships with men who become violent towards her). The problematic consequences of individualising these issues is that they are moved outside the realms of justice and into the remit of benevolent welfare – a system which, as we have already seen in the stories of Lily and Natalie, is replete with institutional ableism and further violence. These conceptions of disability justice, grounded as they are in exclusion or exceptionality, link to presumptions about disability as an individual pathology, or as Riddle (2014, p. 96) suggests, 'as residing in the individual and not as a consequence of the political, social and economic conditions'.

Flynn (2015) importantly recognises that, because of the diversity of the disability experience, there is a need to draw on theories of justice from an intersectional standpoint. However, as Hill Collins and Bilge (2016, p. 30) note, 'social justice may be intersectionality's most contentious core idea'. While intersectional frameworks may have *prima facie* usefulness in explaining how the organisation of power impacts on disability as an identity category, one criticism of the approach concerns the overuse of personal identity as a category of analysis and the consequent underemphasis on structural and particularly material conditions (Hill Collins and Bilge 2016). The complexity inherent in the multiple intersecting domains we see in Lily and Natalie's different trajectories of injustice demonstrates the need for a more nuanced examination of disability as part of intersectionality that, as Erevelles (2011, p. 26) argues, should focus on 'the actual social and economic conditions that impact disabled people's lives, and that are concurrently mediated by the politics of race, ethnicity, gender, sexuality and nation'. The operationalisation of a justice-based approach to gendered disability violence has to date been beset by the relative absence of a more inclusive account grounded in the experiences of the diversity of disabled women and so has fallen short in considering or accounting for the possibility of divergent (un)justice outcomes.

Here, the issue of an accurate characterisation of the experiences of impairment and disability is central, since the judgements made about the causes of disability, about the meaning of the concept, and about the factors to hold responsible for the experience of disability have profound consequences for the direction pursued by advocates, policymakers, politicians and the courts (Rioux 1997). Disability studies as a discipline has, since the 1980s, debated the relative importance of key concepts such as impairment and disability, identity, gender, geopolitical positioning and the relations between them for an overarching conceptual model of disability (Goodley 2011). Early ascendant social models emerged in response to traditional medicalisation and tragedy views and positioned disability as a socially constructed category shaped by differential responses to non-normative bodies and minds (Corker and French 1999). Critique of this somewhat overly simplistic position has emerged in more recent times to challenge thinking about the role of impairment, of identity and of the intersectional operations of social inequality.

Of particular relevance to an examination of dichotomous unjust outcomes for women who are subject to gendered disability violence is consideration of those inside and outside recognised disability identity categories. For Lily, the spatial location of her violent experiences as having occurred within a 'disability' setting allows for some limited recognition within justice responses, where we see her experience recognised although ultimately excluded from successful prosecution: 'The police were surprised as they absolutely believed her and could not understand why the case wasn't prosecuted.' Natalie's impairments are differently entangled. Here we observe the impact of 'corrosive disadvantage' (Wolff and de-Shalit 2007), whereby several dimensions of risk and disadvantage cluster together and compound one other (p. 9). In Natalie's experience we observe that the presence of complex social disadvantage yields further disadvantage, particularly in the recognition of justice claims related to violence – including interpersonal, systemic and institutional violence. This compounding violence highlights the harmful implications of formulating understandings of disability or gender via pure social categorisation as a positive identity position, which may or may not be adopted by any one individual or recognised by any one institution. Notions of vulnerability and negative identities associated with offending, danger and risk, even when disability is present, may be politically and technically distanced from positive justice claims, reinforcing conceptions of the 'deserving' disabled person as the only kind of disabled 'victim' in need of justice. This is in contrast to the 'unworthy' whose impairments are entangled with corrosive social disadvantage and whose claims to disability identity are overshadowed by those of offender, provocateur, drug user, bad mother and so on. This bifurcation excludes many actual experiences of gendered disability violence and poses significant challenges to an inclusive practical justice.

Mandates for practical justice in gendered disability violence

I will now return to Lily and Natalie in order to examine what a practical justice approach might mean for them and for women experiencing gendered disability violence. At its most rudimentary, their negative experiences suggest two key mandates which a practical justice approach must address: (1) recognition of injustice, and (2) redress of injustice. Importantly, these two are intertwined in the sense that failure to address recognition necessarily results in the failure of redress.

Recognition of injustice

The first mandate in addressing the practicality of ensuring justice for women experiencing gendered disability violence is to enable *individual, institutional* and *systemic* recognition of injustice. Lily's experience of gendered disability violence is recognised at the individual level by Lily and those around her. The presence of a supportive and affirming family in which Lily's parents are attuned to her communication of the violence she experienced – 'my daughter is very clear and knowledgeable about not only the sexual abuse but also the decisions made by those in control concerning every aspect of her life' – and their willingness to support and advocate for recognition via police and further legal intervention acts as a protective factor for recognition on an individual level. That 'the police ... absolutely believed her' similarly indicates that with sensitive and skilled investigative expertise, individual law enforcement officers are also able to recognise and affirm experiences of gendered disability violence.

Although we know little about the actions of the disability service at the disclosure of Lily's experience, recent evidence from Australia's *Royal Commission into Institutional Responses to Childhood Sexual Abuse* (2017), various national and state enquiries into violence and abuse in disability settings, and similar commissions of enquiry in other Western liberal democracies[2] reveal an enduring legacy of institutional cultures of cover-up and inaction in the face of damning evidence of widespread violence and abuse in disability settings. The lack of strong mechanisms for oversight, reporting and sanction work against the practical justice responses that require recognition of institutional responsibility for the provision of safe social care environments. So while individual recognition may be a positive for at least some aspects of practical justice, the absence of interconnected accountability at the institutional level runs the risk of reinforcing the tendencies of neoliberal and market mechanisms of social care and of justice to continue to hold the individual responsible for their own wellbeing.

Systemically, Lily's experience is one of denial of justice. Despite police recognition of her experience of violence, they 'could not understand why the case wasn't prosecuted', suggesting a failure of legal processes of prosecution which are premised on the likelihood of evidence leading to a conviction. So while Lily's own information to police left no doubt in their minds as to the veracity of her claims, she fails higher-order tests of evidence to be used to obtain a prosecution within formal legal processes. This phenomenon is well recognised in relation to women with intellectual disability particularly, where systemic assumptions regarding the reliability of such individuals as witnesses and the unwillingness or inability of the legal system to provide support and accommodations to enable women to provide their evidence in court (Keilty and Connelly 2001) works actively against the recognition of their justice claims. There is also a wholesale failure of recognition of the systemic risk factors associated with Lily's spatial location at the time of the violence as within a 'disability' context. As argued earlier in this chapter, it is known that closed environments such as social care, health and corrective facilities actively operate to expose women with disability to gendered disability violence by virtue of their entrenched power relations of care and dependency. There is also ambivalence at work here in the interconnections between the individual, institutional and the systemic, where Lily's institutional location within a disability service provides for a recognition that disability, as an individual attribute, is present for her and therefore informs, for example, police actions in response to her experience. At the same time, however, the fact that disability spaces themselves expose women to a higher likelihood of gendered disability violence goes unacknowledged. Addressing this obscuring of individual, institutional and systemic interconnections requires an integrated framework of recognition to underpin practical justice responses to gendered disability violence.

Natalie's experience of recognition requires a more complex evaluation, which rests on moving beyond simple conceptions of disability to examine its entanglement in a web of corrosive disadvantage. At the individual level, Natalie's experience of homelessness, criminalisation, serial violence, hospitalisation, incarceration and child removal highlights the absence of effective informal supports that might include family and community. The entanglement of intergenerational disadvantage, gender, disability and family violence, and care and dependency relationships, which are mutually negatively reinforcing, mark Natalie out as a highly vulnerable young woman. Yet institutional responses are deferred to agencies of surveillance and control. Rather than recognition of her experiences as shaped by the presence of disability, her multiple negative labels of offender, perpetrator, drug user or bad mother give rise to what Dodds (2014, p. 197) has termed 'pathogenic vulnerability'. This calls attention to the ways in which for Natalie, socio-institutional structures themselves generate dependency, which exacerbates individual vulnerability where 'institutional arrangements fail to address the complex relationships between dependency and vulnerability' (p. 196). A practical justice response that takes account of this positioning and specifically recognises the presence of multiple compounding social disadvantage and disability as a key marker for a higher likelihood of injustice is needed.

Natalie's experience of justice is characterised by systematic entrenchment in negative processes and spaces of punishment, where her particular forms of individual need are stigmatised. Overt institutional violence is wrought by this dependence on systemic 'care'. The failure of individual responses of support and justice – for example for her early experiences of sexual and family violence – or the failure of educational, child protection or youth and adult justice institutions to recognise and respond to her own violence and self-harm as symptomatic of deeper trauma, propel her into a cycle of serial exclusion from support services, where the lack of coherent institutional response ultimately circumscribes any possibility for further forms of justice to be practically enacted. Natalie's experience of multiple institutional failure leads to her subsequent entrenchment in a revolving-door system of institutional containment as the default response, itself characterised by further violence, which is very often obscured from public view. A recent Human Rights Watch (2018) report highlights the dehumanisation and brutality to which women with disability in Australian prisons are subject. Ultimately Natalie becomes what Starr Sered and Norton-Hawk (2014) term an 'institutional captive', where her experiences of the welfare/penal/medical/ disability support system act as one interlocking metasystem. In practical justice terms, addressing the web of individual, institutional and systemic disavowal that Natalie experiences requires an operational recognition that access to justice is conditioned by a complexity of factors, which for some women begin to compound from early life. The largely a-historical and a-political point-in-time interventions that characterise various processes of justice result in the systematic suppression of consideration of the multiple and compounding systemic factors which naturalise disadvantage and essentialise disability. A practical justice response must take as its starting point recognition of these complex fundamentals of gendered disability violence and demand coherence in institutional responses, which include spaces of safety, trauma-informed practice and systemic monitoring and accountability.

Redress of injustice

The disjuncture between recognition of injustice and its systemic redress speaks to the deeply ableist assumptions within processes and systems of justice which, while perhaps enabling some individual recognition, as we see in Lily's experience, still fail to provide redress via inclusive approaches which acknowledge, enable and support. For Lily, there is a failure of the mechanism to convert recognition into redress, while for Natalie even the most basic recognition appears beyond the capacity of systems of justice to deliver. These failures represent a form of institutional violence in which the lack of redress further traumatises disabled women and de-authorises their justice claims.

Traditional responses to gendered disability violence have been premised on the notion of protection, an accepted and long-standing trope associated with women with intellectual disability in particular. But as we can see in the experiences of Lily, protectionist approaches – which, for instance, might assume that the trauma of giving evidence in court against a perpetrator results in inadequate testimony and further upset – are the ultimate denial of a central tenet of practical justice: namely, to have one's claims heard and responded to. For Natalie, where complex social disadvantage is also present, no such protection is afforded. Rather the result is an intensification of vulnerability, stigmatisation and criminalisation – re-entrenching corrosive disadvantage and leading to increasingly perverse and damagingly violent outcomes.

Justice operates at conceptual and theoretical levels as well as operationally through various frameworks, including human rights, jurisdictional legal structures, participation in justice systems and processes of representation in the legislative sphere in which justice claims are debated. Flynn (2015) (drawing on and adding to the work of Bahdi [2007]) provides a useful framework for conceptualising forms of redress for the types of societal disadvantage that shape disabled women's experiences of violence. These centre on four forms of access to justice: procedural, substantive, symbolic and participatory (p. 13). Specifically, the development of clear mandates for practical redress for the injustice associated with gendered disability violence requires attention to processes associated with: the *procedural*, in recognising the nature and quality of encounters for women with disability within legal institutions such as courts and tribunals; the *substantive*, in the legal rules and principles which shape decisions made about those who make a justice claim; the *symbolic*, in the inclusion of women with disability as equal citizens in legal regimes; and the *participatory*, where disabled women are included and contribute to civil society, legal and human rights debates about issues which affect their lives.

Conclusions

The risks for gendered disability violence in domestic, community and institutional settings is being increasingly recognised, but entrenched institutional ableism is not. Without proper deliberation and understanding of the multiple and diverse experiences of disability or the multiple other issues implicated in disability, we will continue to condone systems which flagrantly make exceptions of disability in the recognition and redress of gendered disability violence, through a system which 'permits' and 'excuses' the infringement of the human rights to safety, bodily integrity and equality before the law. If our responses are to be 'just', they cannot simply be about recognition of a diagnosis and the application of accommodations – as if it were that simple. Instead, the intersection of gender, disability and violence – and the multiple domains of power they entail – call for a more sophisticated form of analysis that enables us to protect and promote the rights and safety of women in all their diversity. Ultimately, addressing issues of gendered disability violence is one of equitable access to justice.

Notes

1 Case study drawn from the longitudinal administrative linked dataset compiled from Australian Research Council (ARC) Linkage project, 'People with Mental Health Disorders and Cognitive Disabilities in the Criminal Justice System (CJS) in NSW', University of NSW – Chief Investigators E. Baldry, L. Dowse and I Webster. www.mhdcd.unsw.edu.au. Ethics approval was obtained from all the relevant ethics bodies, including from the University of New South Wales Human Research Ethics Committee.

2 See, in Australia: Community Affairs References Committee (2015); Finance and
   Public Administration References Committee (2015); Parliament of Victoria
   Family and Community Development Committee (2014); UK: Bubb (2014);
   Ireland: National Disability Authority (2013); Canada: DisAbled Women's
   Network, Canada (2011); New Zealand: Mirfin-Veitch and Conder (2017).

References

Bahdi, R., 2007. *Background Paper on Women's Access to Justice in the MENA Region.* International Development Research Centre (IDRC), Women's Rights and Citizenship (WRC) Program, and the Middle East Regional Office (MERO), Middle East and North African (MENA) Regional Consultation, 9–11 December 2007, Cairo, Egypt. Available from: www.uwindsor.ca/law/rbahdi/sites/uwindsor.ca.law.rbahdi/files/womens_access_to_justice_in_mena-bahdi_en.pdf [Accessed 15 February 2018].

Bubb, S., 2014. *Winterborne View – Time for Change.* Transforming Care and Commissioning Steering Group. Available from: www.england.nhs.uk/wp-content/uploads/2014/11/transforming-commissioning-services.pdf [Accessed 23 September 2015].

Chenoweth, L., 1997. Violence and Women with Disabilities: Silence and Paradox. In: S. Cook and J. Bessant, eds, *Women's Encounters: Australian Experiences.* Thousand Oaks, CA: Sage, 21–39.

Clark, H. and Fileborn, B., 2011. *Responding to Women's Experiences of Sexual Assault in Institutional and Care Settings.* Melbourne: Australian Centre for the Study of Sexual Assault. Available from: https://aifs.gov.au/ [Accessed 12 September 2017].

Commonwealth of Australia, 2010. *National Plan to Reduce Violence against Women and their Children 2010–2022.* Canberra: Council of Australian Governments.

Community Affairs References Committee, 2015. *Violence, Abuse and Neglect against People with Disability in Institutional and Residential Settings, Including the Gender and Age Related Dimensions, and the Particular Situation of Aboriginal and Torres Strait Islander People with Disability, and Culturally and Linguistically Diverse People with Disability.* Canberra: Commonwealth of Australia. Available from: www.aph.gov.au/Parliamentary_Business/Committees/Senate/Community_Affairs/Violence_abuse_neglect/Report [Accessed 6 March 2016].

Corker, M. and French, S., 1999. Reclaiming Discourse in Disability Studies. In: M. Corker and S. French, eds, *Disability Discourse.* Buckingham: Open University Press, 1–12.

Convention on the Rights of Persons with Disabilities (CRPD), 2013. *Committee on the Rights of Persons with Disabilities: Concluding Observations on the Initial Report of Australia, Adopted by the Committee at Its Tenth Session (2–13 September 2013).* Available from: http://docstore.ohchr.org/SelfServices [Accessed 10 August 2017].

Dillon, J., 2010. *Violence against People with Cognitive Impairments.* Office of the Public Advocate. Available from: www.publicadvocate.vic.gov.au/research/255/ [Accessed 13 February 2018].

DisAbled Women's Network Canada, 2011. *Women with Disabilities and Abuse: Access to Supports.* Canadian Women's Foundation. Available from: www.canadian-women.org/wp-content/uploads/2017/09/PDF-VP-Resource-DAWN-RAFH-Canada-Focus-Groups-WWD_201.pdf [Accessed 23 September 2017].

Dodds, S., 2014. Dependence, Care, and Vulnerability. In: C. Mackenzie, W. Rogers and S. Dodds, eds, *Vulnerability: New Essays in Ethics and Feminist Philosophy*. New York: Oxford University Press, 204–221.

Dowse, L., Dean, K., Trofimovs, J. and Tzoumakis, S., 2015. *People with Complex Needs who are the Victims of Crime: Building Evidence for Responsive Support*. Report for the NSW Department of Justice. Available from: www.victimsclearinghouse.nsw.gov.au/ Documents/People_with_Complex_Needs_and_Crime_Victimisation_Final_ Report_Jan_2015.pdf [Accessed 1 March 2018].

Dowse, L., Soldatic, K., Didi, A., Frohmader, C. and van Toorn, G., 2013. *Stop the Violence: Addressing Violence against Women and Girls with Disabilities in Australia, Background Paper*. Hobart: Women with Disabilities Australia. Available from: http://wwda.org.au [Accessed 12 November 2017].

Dowse, L., Soldatic, K., Spangaro, J. and van Toorn, G., 2016. Mind the Gap: The Extent of Violence against Women with Disabilities in Australia. *Australian Journal of Social Issues*, 51 (3), 341–359.

Erevelles, N., 2011. *Disability and Difference in Global Contexts: Enabling a Transformative Body Politics*. New York: Palgrave Macmillan.

Finance and Public Administration References Committee, 2015. *Domestic Violence in Australia*. Canberra: Commonwealth of Australia. Available from: www.aph. gov.au/Parliamentary_Business/Committees/Senate/Finance_and_Public_ Administration/Domestic_Violence/Report [Accessed 9 September 2016].

Flynn, E., 2015. *Disabled Justice? Access to Justice and the UN Convention of the Rights of Persons with Disabilities*. Abingdon: Routledge.

Goodley, D., 2011. *Disability Studies: An Interdisciplinary Introduction*. London: Sage.

Hill Collins, P. and Bilge, S., 2016. *Intersectionality*. Malden, MA: Polity Press.

Human Rights Watch, 2018. *'I Needed Help, Instead I Was Punished': Abuse and Neglect of Prisoners with Disabilities in Australia*. Human Rights Watch. Available from: www.hrw.org/report/2018/02/06/i-needed-help-instead-i-was-punished/abuse- and-neglect-prisoners-disabilities [Accessed 7 February 2018].

International Network of Women with Disabilities (INWWD), 2013. *Interdependence: Including Women with Disabilities in the Agenda of the Women's Movement – Our Fears, Realities, Hopes and Dreams*. Submission by Myra Kovary, Coordinator of INWWD, to the Half-Day of General Discussion on Women and Girls with Disabilities at the 9th Session of the UNCRPD, 17 April 2013. Available from: www.ohchr.org/EN/ HRBodies/CRPD/Pages/DGD17April2013.aspx [Accessed 14 November 2017].

Keilty, J. and Connelly, G., 2001. Making a Statement: An Exploratory Study of Barriers Facing Women with an Intellectual Disability when Making a Statement about Sexual Assault to Police. *Disability & Society*, 16 (2), 273–291.

Lund, E. M., 2012. Violence against People with Disabilities: New Developments and Important Implications. *Spotlight on Disability Newsletter*, December. Available from: www.apa.org/pi/disability/resources/publications/newsletter/2012/12/ disabilities-violence.aspx [Accessed 16 November 2017].

Lykkee, N., 2010. *Feminist Studies: A Guide to Intersectional Theory, Methodology and Writing*. London: Routledge.

Meekosha, H. and Dowse, L., 1997. Enabling Citizenship: Gender, Disability and Citizenship. *Feminist Review*, 57, 49–72.

Mirfin-Veitch, B. and Conder, J., 2017. *'Institutions are Places of Abuse': The Experiences of Disabled Children and Adults in State Care between 1950–1992*. Dunedin: The Donald Beasley Institute.

National Disability Authority, 2013. *Domestic Violence and Abuse against People with Disabilities.* Joint Oireachtas Committee on Justice, Defence and Equality. Available from: http://nda.ie/nda-files/Paper-by-the-National-Disability-Authority-to-Joint-Oireachtas-Committee-on-Justice-Defence-and-Equality-May-20131.pdf [Accessed 8 September 2017].

Nussbaum, M. C., 2011. *Creating Capabilities.* Cambridge, MA: Harvard University Press.

Ortoleva, S. and Lewis. H., 2012. Forgotten Sisters – A Report on Violence against Women with Disabilities: An Overview of Its Nature, Scope, Causes and Consequences. *Northeastern University School of Law Research Paper No. 104–2012.* Available from: https://ssrn.com/abstract=2133332 [Accessed 8 September 2017].

Parliament of Victoria Family and Community Development Committee, 2014. *Inquiry into Abuse in Disability Services Final Report.* Melbourne: Parliament of Victoria. Available from: www.parliament.vic.gov.au/file_uploads/FCDC_Inquiry_into_abuse_in_disability_services_HtW37zgf.pdf [Accessed 12 August 2017].

People with Disability Australia, n.d. *A History of the Disability Rights Movement in Australia.* Available from: www.pwd.org.au/student-section/history-of-disability-rights-movement-in-australia.html [Accessed 12 March 2018].

Price-Kelly, S. and Attard, M., 2010. *Accommodating Violence: The Experience of Domestic Violence and People with Disability Living in Licensed Boarding Houses.* Sydney: People with Disabilities Australia. Available from: www.pwd.org.au/ [Accessed 13 October 2017].

Riddle, C. A., 2014. *Disability and Justice: The Capabilities Approach in Practice.* Lanham, MD: Lexington Books.

Rioux, M. H., 1997. Disability: The Place of Judgement in a World of Fact. *Journal of Intellectual Disability Research,* 41 (2), 102–111.

Robinson, S., 2013. *Preventing the Emotional Abuse and Neglect of People with Intellectual Disability: Stopping Insult and Injury.* London: Jessica Kingsley Publishers.

Sherry, M., 2000. Hate Crimes against Disabled People. *Social Alternatives,* 19 (4), 23–30.

Starr Sered, S. and Norton-Hawk, M., 2014. *Can't Catch a Break: Gender, Jail, Drugs, and the Limits of Personal Responsibility.* Berkeley: University of California Press.

Stathopoulos, M., 2012. *Addressing Women's Victimisation Histories in Custodial Settings.* Melbourne: Australian Centre for the Study of Sexual Assault.

Wolff, J. and de-Shalit, A., 2007. *Disadvantage.* Oxford: Oxford University Press.

Women with Disabilities Australia (WWDA), 2011. *Submission to the UN Analytical Study on Violence against Women with Disabilities.* Rosny Park: WWDA. Available from: http://wwda.org.au/ [Accessed 24 September 2017].

Chapter 4

Supporting mental health in low-income communities

Implications for justice and equity

Felicity Thomas and Lorraine Hansford

Introduction

Mental health problems are currently viewed as constituting one of the greatest burdens on global health and wellbeing (WHO 2017). Recent years have witnessed a marked rise in mental health diagnoses and in the prescribing of mental health treatments across much of the economically developed world. Diagnosis for depressive disorders and anxiety disorders (common mental disorders) in particular have shown a marked rise in recent years. Although depression can and does affect people from all backgrounds, the risk of becoming depressed is increased by poverty, unemployment and other challenging life circumstances (WHO 2017).

Set against a broader background of austerity and ongoing welfare reforms in countries such as the UK, the chapter explores the paradox between growing equity in access to mental health diagnosis and treatment and the high level of discontent and injustice being experienced by those living with poverty-related distress. Drawing on findings from DeStress (see http://destressproject.org.uk), a two-and-a-half-year study in England, the chapter draws out two key, inter-related ways in which forms of injustice impact upon people in low-income communities: first, providing an overview of the ways in which experiences of poverty and engagement with the welfare system can engender and exacerbate underlying vulnerabilities to mental distress; and second, focusing on the wellbeing implications of medicalising poverty-related distress. Particular attention is given to the relevance, effectiveness and ethics of current treatment options and their implications in terms of equitable service provision and support.

Mental health and treatment justice

The past decade has seen an unprecedented rise in the administration and use of pharmaceutical treatments for mental health. In Australia, anti-depressants are now the most commonly used medications, being taken by 10 per cent of the adult population at a rate that has more than doubled since 2000 (Davey and Chanen 2016). A similar picture can be seen in the USA, where there has also been a marked increase in long-term use of these medications (Mojtabai and Olfson 2014). In England, the number of antidepressant items prescribed more than doubled from 33.7 million in 2006 to 64.7 million in 2016 (NHS Digital 2017). Recent analyses demonstrate high levels of prescribing and use of psychoactive drugs in low-income communities (Anderson *et al.* 2009, Lewer *et al.* 2015, EXASOL 2017), with a parallel upsurge in the availability and promotion of talking therapies. Indeed, in England, where the government has committed strongly to the Improving Access to Psychological Therapies (IAPT) pro-gramme, over 900,000 patients a year had been seen by 2008, with plans to expand this to upward of 1.5 million a year by 2020 (Clark 2011).

One reading of these trends is that government-provided mental health services have successfully challenged the inverse care law, by ensuring that widely recommended treatments are available to all who need them. In England, this stance appears to be backed up by an array of government policy committing to move towards parity of esteem between mental and physical health in terms of access to services, quality of care and allocation of resources (NHS 2015, Parkin and Powell 2017). This form of 'treatment justice' may be a sign that mental health stigma has decreased, and that more people now feel comfortable asking for help for depression and anxiety.

However, it may also be argued that these changes are part of an increasing trend towards the pathologisation of everyday stresses, a situation that in turn incites stigma and medicalisation, and that absolves those with power from taking responsibility for the injustices caused by ongoing economic, social and health inequalities.

Poverty, pathology and welfare

Much recent thinking around mental illness has been influenced by the dominance of medical guidelines, such as the Diagnostic and Statistical Manual (DSM) and the International Classification of Diseases (ICD), whose classifications and categories set boundaries on what should and should not be defined as 'normal' behaviour. Yet the authority of such guidelines, and in particular, the DSM V, have been widely criticised (see for example, Dowrick and Frances 2013) for expanding the boundaries of what counts as mental disorder so far that emotions such as sadness and grief have become recast as forms of clinical depression.

In a situation where what would once have been considered unexceptional and expected reactions to common life stresses can lead to diagnosis with a mental health 'condition', it is important to consider how poverty and deprivation – known to constitute key factors in the creation and exacerbation of mental distress – intersect with psychiatric diagnosis and mental health treatment. This is particularly apposite in the context of economic austerity, where strategies to reform the system of welfare entitlement may impact on those aimed at supporting mental health and wellbeing, and where the chances of poverty-related distress being diagnosed and treated as mental *illness* are now extremely high.

If mental health diagnosis and treatment means that people experiencing mental ill health are receiving appropriate support, this 'pathologisation of everything' (Conrad 2007) may rightly be seen as an important step forward for healthcare justice and parity. However, in situations where people's social identity and access to welfare support are increasingly and intrinsically connected to their health status and their ability to evidence sickness, this situation also raises a wide range of important ethical debates over the role that welfare reforms play in exacerbating distress, and the ways that pathologisation and medicalisation intersect with poverty and disadvantage. This in turn calls into question the relevance, effectiveness and even potential for harm of the dominant treatment options that are being promoted under the auspices of supporting and enhancing people's mental health.

The pathological self

Associations between poverty and mental ill health are well established, with most explanations expounding a two-way process or a vicious cycle in which poverty may be seen to cause mental ill health, and mental ill health may be seen to lead to, or to exacerbate, poverty. Yet, while research on deprivation and mental health draws attention to the potentially distressing effects of living in poverty, there is little conclusive evidence about the nature of the relationship between the factors at play, nor what this might mean in terms of people's lived experience, or the appropriateness of mental health treatments available to them. A key issue here relates to the ways in which efforts to promote mental health, and much of the literature upon which these are based, remain focused at the level of the individual, meaning that mental health concerns become framed as a pathological problem of the 'self' (Busfield 2011). This has two major implications. First, a stance that is psychologically and behaviourally focused will inevitably reinforce a level of individualised blame and reiterate stereotypical assumptions about the behaviour of people living in deprived circumstances, leading to the re-inscription of deficits-based thinking that sees distressed people who are living in poverty as somehow deficient and in need of 'correction' through medical or therapeutic intervention. Second, by pathologising individuals as having a distinct and categorisable 'defect' within their brain or psychological functioning, mental health is viewed and treated in a disempowering apolitical vacuum, where the root causes of deprivation and social injustice that are known to sustain poverty and underpin the erosion of wellbeing become obscured (Shaw and Taplin 2007, Friedli 2013).

This is especially pertinent in the current economic climate, where notions of self and self-responsibility have been progressively amplified through neo-liberally oriented government policies to encourage the uptake of employment and to restrict access to welfare entitlements. For over three decades, successive British governments have been claiming that the social security system has 'lost its way', and that large-scale reform is needed to abolish what George Osborne as Chancellor described as an entrenched 'something for nothing culture' (Blackburn 2013) in which people in receipt of benefits 'shamelessly' expect to be provided for while expecting others to go out to work.

As Walker (2014) has argued, this kind of vitriolic rhetoric has popular appeal, particularly in times of austerity, and, by rendering 'welfare' as a term of abuse, has facilitated a range of reforms that have led to wide-scale reductions in welfare entitlements across the UK. Amongst other things, this includes a cap on the benefits available to an individual or household, the introduction of a controversial 'simplified' payment system through the roll-out of 'Universal Credit', and the imposition of the 'bedroom tax', whereby people living in social housing that is deemed to surpass their basic needs now have to pay for any 'spare' bedrooms within the property.

Importantly, these welfare reform strategies, as well as popular contemporary media, and encounters with key service providers such as Jobcentres (see Friedli and Stearn 2015), are imbued with moralising narratives that promote the idea that individuals and households facing challenging circumstances should have been more 'responsible' in their actions to protect and enhance their health and wellbeing, and should have acted as 'good' and 'entrepreneurial' citizens (Crawford 2006, Ayo 2012) to maximise personal and societal interests while relieving the burden on the welfare system (Lupton 1995, Leichter 1997). Such thinking implies that those who are living in challenging or precarious circumstances have brought this upon themselves through irresponsible decision-making and actions. As a result, those in receipt of welfare support are now widely and publicly condemned as undeserving 'scroungers', unless they can provide convincing evidence that there are exceptional health circumstances that preclude them from employment. Indeed, recent research has found a hardening of attitudes against those in receipt of welfare support in the UK (NatCen 2013), as well as increased feelings of shame, stigma and disassociation within low-income communities themselves (Shildrick and MacDonald 2013).

Welfare and employment

Against this background, the DeStress project, which employed a range of qualitative methods (focus groups, interviews, conversation analysis of video-recorded GP–patient consultations), aimed to investigate the impacts of austerity and welfare reform on mental health in low-income communities; the relevance and effectiveness of current treatment options; and the challenges facing general practitioners (GPs) working with low-income patients experiencing poverty-related distress.[1]

Far from constituting the 'easy option' that is so often portrayed within government rhetoric and popular media, findings from the project consistently emphasise the high levels of anxiety and stress that result not only from the challenges of poverty, but from engagement within the welfare system itself. The need to attend regular appointments (usually dependent on unreliable public transport), to provide sufficient evidence of job-seeking (requiring access to computer and Internet) for limited and usually precarious work opportunities, to keep in line with the array of changes to benefits and associated rules that have been enforced in recent years, to deal with and challenge what many describe as frequent under- or delayed payments or benefits sanctions, to be shown to be 'bettering' yourself through voluntary work placements and to display the necessary 'work ready' psychology (see Friedli and Stearn 2015) to convince benefits advisors of your credibility were just some of the challenges that people felt added to the stresses of their lives.

Katherine,[2] for example, a full-time volunteer worker at her local community centre, was sanctioned in 2016 for missing a meeting after the Jobcentre failed to alert her to a changed appointment time, meaning that she received no payments at all for eight weeks. Yet as her account makes clear, this was just one of her many experiences of missing or chasing up unpaid benefits:

> I can spend hours and hours on the phone trying to sort the problem out so we actually will get paid. I mean, on average, out of a two-month period at least three payments out of the four I will have to ring them up to chase my benefit payment so that we actually get the money [...] I'm very lucky 'cos our daughter has a contract phone, which has minutes, so she will usually allow me to use her phone to ring ... I haven't had any credit on my mobile for nearly two years, 'cos I just cannot afford to put credit on [...] it gets me down, and after being on the phone for so long and having to go through it so many times, you know, I do get very, very disheartened with it. I know for a fact that, I mean, my husband with all his mental health problems and everything, I know, he couldn't do it. I know he couldn't do it. He couldn't cope with it. And there are a lot of people out there who can't because before now I have actually had people come up to me, where I volunteer, asking me to make these phone calls for them because they just can't cope with doing it, you know.

Welfare entitlement is also increasingly assessed via the possession of a legitimately certified 'disability', with previous health assessments no longer deemed as credible evidence to support existing claims. At face value, the underlying aim to 'encourage' people away from welfare and into employment is perhaps not in itself unreasonable, since there is ample evidence of the mental-health-related benefits of work (Modini *et al.* 2016). Yet, recent years have witnessed increasing levels of poverty within working households in the UK (Tinson *et al.* 2016), with work-related stress and poor mental wellbeing being closely associated with the kinds of precarious and often low-paid employment commonly available to those facing situations of hardship. Indeed, a recent report from Ireland (see Bobek *et al.* 2018) has shown clearly that precarious work is often associated with narrowly defined contracts and unpredictable hours, and can lead to a range of obstacles for people trying to establish families, or to secure loans, mortgages, or even to obtain rented accommodation. Furthermore, precarious work has been found to have negative impacts on both physical and mental health, which is in turn particularly problematic when people have no recourse to sick leave. Thus, while policies that encourage people to take up work may be empowering in some instances, evidence suggests they frequently push people towards situations that may ultimately reduce, rather than improve, their quality of life.

Assessing the legitimacy of people's welfare claims also means that people living with chronic physical and/or mental health problems are now required to undergo more frequent medical assessments to decide their suitability for work. This procedure is undertaken by private companies that usually have no prior relationship with, nor insight into, the broader context and realities of an individual's life. For participants in the DeStress project who found themselves in this situation, the medical reassessment process was extremely traumatic and morally undermining, especially when one's poor health status was questioned and de-legitimised during the assessment process. Participants in this situation explained how repeated medical assessment could greatly exacerbate mental distress, and lead to adverse economic repercussions when doubts about a person's claims resulted in their benefits being cut or withdrawn. Terry's case was typical of the kinds of stress and injustice caused by medical reassessment:

> Terry (58) lives with his wife (50) in an economically deprived area of Plymouth. Despite being unable to read or write, Terry worked for around 20 years as a manual labourer and barman before being made redundant. Although he has since undertaken short bouts of work, his poor health means he has been unable to find secure employment during the past two decades. He explained that during this time, he has suffered from long bouts of depression and has multiple physical health issues that impede his breathing and heart functioning. In 2017, Terry received notice that he was required to attend a medical review procedure where, despite his age, health status and the support

of his GP, he was reassessed as being 'fit for work'. At that point, Terry lost his right to Employment Support Allowance, leaving the couple to survive on £105 a week. From this, they pay all their bills, and are liable for a £25-a-week 'bedroom tax' because the local authority has been unable to relocate them to a smaller property. Terry attends regular appointments with his GP where he gets sick notes that exempt him from having to evidence job-seeking. However, this is a time-limited 'solution' and the uncertainty of his situation and the couple's ongoing poverty is a major cause of distress that intensifies their already poor health and wellbeing.

As Terry's case demonstrates, poverty and the demands of the welfare process can exacerbate vulnerabilities to intense distress and severe mental health issues within low-income communities. However, in a situation in which welfare requirements mean that poverty-related distress is increasingly medicalised, it is also important to consider whether the support available to people through mental health diagnosis and treatment necessarily acts to support equity or may, in cases, actually create injustice.

The medicalisation of distress

Research has shown that people in low-income communities face a range of socioculturally determined issues that deter them from seeking formal help for mental distress (Clement *et al.* 2015). For some of the male participants in the DeStress study, this deterrent was associated with identity, pride and social status, with help-seeking seen to engender shame and weakness. For others, there were more practical concerns relating to the logistics of travel and childcare, as well as a palpable fear amongst many parents who felt that asking for help for mental health and wellbeing-related issues would lead to their children being taken into the care of social services.

Despite the challenges people face in seeking support, it is clear from national prescribing data that many people from low-income communities *do* at some point in time turn to health professionals to seek support for mental distress (NHS Digital 2017). This may indicate that the person understands their distress through a medical framework, and accepts that they require some form of medically focused treatment. However, in a situation in which large-scale and ongoing resource cuts in the UK voluntary sector mean that GPs are often the only people left that people feel able to go to for help, and where GPs act as the main conduit for the administration of sick notes (now tellingly renamed 'fitness for work' notes) needed by people to evidence their ill health, the picture is often much more complex.

Whatever the situation, formal responses to mental health problems remain limited to two main forms of support and treatment: talking therapies and/or antidepressant medications. While prescribing data imply that access to these treatments has improved in recent years, work carried out as part of the DeStress project demonstrates how both options may in fact shape experiences of, and responses to, mental health and wellbeing in ways that exacerbate rather than alleviate harm and injustice.

Talking therapies

In the past decade, considerable emphasis has been placed on the potential for non-medical interventions as a first line of support for people diagnosed with low-level depression and anxiety. Despite the Improving Access to Psychological Therapies (IAPT) programme being widely heralded as a successful non-medical intervention, such services are currently delivered and evaluated through a 'one-size-fits-all' approach that disregards social and economic variation in need and provision in order to meet standardised targets around notions of 'improvement' and 'recovery', and aims to achieve this within the limits of six to eight sessions of group or individual counselling.

Central to this provision is a generally accepted requirement amongst health and service providers for people to self-refer to IAPT as a necessary 'first step to recovery'. Yet findings from DeStress indicate that a range of factors deter people from low-income groups self-referring for this kind of therapeutic support service. GPs interviewed and observed repeatedly emphasised the ease with which people could self-refer, and the need for patients to 'take responsibility' for themselves. However, almost all patients interviewed who had been referred to IAPT stressed the mental and logistical difficulties they faced doing this. Indeed, for some patients, the giving of the IAPT leaflet constituted a symbolic dismissal that undermined and delegitimised their concerns:

> They gave me a self-referral thing to [local IAPT service] and like, okay, if I can't even pay my bills and I can't even like post a letter on time, then how am I going to, you know, do a self-referral to [local IAPT service]? [...] If you don't pay your water, you got no electric, no gas, how can you live? But you don't think about that when you're depressed – you're like if somebody else does it for you, you feel better, if somebody posts that letter for you or if somebody pays that bill – I mean I've got bills stacking up and stacking up, letters that I need to answer and it's just not that easy. So they go, 'here, self-referral' and you're like no, that's why I need counselling to get out of this mess.
>
> (Delia)

> It took me a lot to go to my doctor. And when I got there, on the first attempt, they gave me that leaflet. And I was just like, 'I don't –

I didn't come here for a leaflet. I came here for some help [...].' He just sent me away. It was like, 'There you go, there's your leaflet, bye.'

(Jonathan)

Alongside the challenges of self-referral, a reluctance to participate in what some saw as an unhelpful or even an indulgent process of self-reflection was clear. Amongst men in particular, there was an aversion to attending therapy when it was felt that it would focus on addressing their perceived mental pathology rather than help tackle the underlying poverty-related causes of their mental health problems. A common complaint amongst those who did attend IAPT, was that counsellors spent too much time focusing on stressful past events which they felt might explain a person's current mental state – or in cases, made unhelpful and often incorrect assumptions around childhood abuse, which both exacerbated people's upset and their distrust of the service, and failed to support what were often more practical stresses around issues such as debt and poor housing.

Perhaps the biggest issue of concern related to the stepped nature of IAPT support, and the difficulties people in low-income communities experienced accessing what they felt was a level of support appropriate to their needs. In one of the DeStress study sites where the IAPT service was formally assessed as 'failing' in meeting its 'recovery' targets, patients who had completed an initial assessment were then commonly refused access to the service because their needs were considered too high. This, in turn, meant that they were referred back to their GP rather than on to more appropriate specialist care, resulting in patients left churning in the system, often for years, with no recourse to any further support.

Antidepressant medications

Recent analysis demonstrates disproportionately high levels of prescribing and use of psychiatric drugs within low-income communities (Anderson *et al.* 2009, EXASOL 2017). While not disputing that these medications can be useful for some people, growing evidence now shows such drugs to have little or no effect in cases of mild depression, and that use of these medications can carry risks associated with harmful side effects, including increased suicidal thinking, and the potential for adverse interactions with other treatment drugs (Gøtzsche 2015).

Figures from a study in Scotland found that a third of all people taking antidepressants long term had no clinical reason to continue with their treatment (Cruickshank *et al.* 2008). Similarly, a number of DeStress study participants who had sought support from their GP had been surprised to find themselves being prescribed with antidepressants, and felt disappointed that this was the only support available to them. A frequently repeated concern was the readiness with which antidepressants were prescribed, and the lack of information they perceived they had been given on the likely side effects of the medications. While the DeStress data suggest that decisions over treatment are often reached as part of a process of negotiation between GP and patient, there was also evidence to suggest that patients were sometimes prescribed antidepressants despite having stated that this went against their wishes. In some interviews, patients revealed that they collected their prescription and got their medications in order to be seen to be obeying the advice of the GP, but they did not then take them. Participants also identified a lack of information or support to help them to stop taking the medications safely, and it was not uncommon for people to recount their painful experiences of going 'cold turkey' with no advice on how best to manage this.

Findings from DeStress also suggest the paradoxically problematic nature of both poor adherence and long-term antidepressant use within low-income communities. Research in the UK shows that half of all people on antidepressants have been taking them for two years or more (Kendrick 2015), a figure that is almost certainly much higher amongst low-income populations. An increasing body of evidence suggests that rather than treating mental ill health, the long-term use of antidepressants can actually be significantly detrimental to mental health and wellbeing – and that in many cases, long-term use of psychiatric medicines not only exacerbates existing mental health conditions, but may also trigger new ones. Data from a recently published 20-year longitudinal study, for example, show that at each follow-up assessment, people who had taken antipsychotic drugs were significantly more likely to display psychotic symptoms than those who had never taken medications (Harrow et al. 2014). Other research suggests that antidepressants not only have limited effectiveness over placebos, but may also affect people's vulnerability to depression in their future lives (Kirsch et al. 2008).

Originally intending to sample people with a mental health diagnosis within the previous two years, it quickly became clear that for most people in the DeStress study sites, antidepressant use had been ongoing across episodes of distress that had persisted for a long time. Gillian's case illustrated this clearly:

> Gillian (26) has been taking anti-depressant medications on and off for long periods of time over the past decade. Having grown up within a violent household, she left home before completing school, and found herself living with an abusive partner with whom she had her first child. Fearing that her child would be taken away if she approached social services for assistance, she sought help from her GP, who diagnosed her with post-natal depression. She received the same diagnosis after the birth of her following two children. Gillian

recognises that many of her negative thoughts stem from her past experiences, and from the ongoing challenges of living on a very low income. Although she feels that the medications help her to cope with life, she feels that there has been little opportunity to try or even to discuss other options for support. The last time she remembers anyone suggesting alternatives to medications was four years ago, and this was never followed up. While she recognises that GPs have few options available to them to help people experiencing poverty-related distress, she feels strongly that there is an inclination amongst service providers towards 'upping the dose' rather than addressing the wider social issues that people experience.

For Gillian, as for others, antidepressants helped her cope with daily life, yet they did not help to solve the underlying causes of the distress and, for a large proportion of interviewees, their use left them feeling numb and disengaged from those around them. In a situation in which GPs are encouraged by clinical guidelines to reassess treatment decisions only when side effects are palpably detrimental to patient health, when health providers are massively constrained by cuts to resourcing, and when people may assume that they are expected to continue treatment unless otherwise advised, the likelihood of people remaining on antidepressants in the long term becomes increasingly apparent. There is therefore an urgent need for health providers to reassess existing practice with respect to antidepressant prescribing in the UK, both to ensure that medications are being prescribed appropriately and to guarantee that their use is monitored and regularly assessed in light of changing patient circumstances. Failure to do this is not only costly and wasteful in terms of resourcing but is morally and ethically dubious.

Conclusions

Recent years have seen a commitment amongst policymakers in England to increasing parity of esteem between mental and physical healthcare and to make mental health treatment more available to all in need. Yet, as this chapter has argued, there has been inadequate critique of the diagnostic assumptions that underpin the evidence upon which such data and such strategies are based, as well as a lack of consideration of the broader economic and political circumstance in which forms of treatment 'justice' are being administered. This becomes deeply problematic when the distress naturally caused by the challenges of poverty and deprivation is increasingly interpreted as clinical depression requiring medical intervention. Indeed, very real questions around justice are brought to the fore when moralising and stigmatising strategies designed to reform the system of welfare support overlap with and impact on those aimed at supporting mental health and wellbeing.

Far from supporting those most in need, we have shown that the increasingly punitive nature of current welfare reform exacerbates under-lying vulnerabilities to mental distress for many people through the widescale reduction of benefit entitlement, the questioning and de-legitimisation of people's medical or disability status and the dehumanis-ing experience and repercussions of dealing with 'the system' itself. At the same time, current treatment options have been shown to have a range of adverse impacts on health and wellbeing that call claims around treatment justice into question. The use of antidepressant medications can numb the realities of poverty and can help enable people to cope with daily life in austerity Britain – yet for many participants in the DeStress study, their use has led to the long-term use of what are often stigmatised, potentially inef-fective and even harmful medications, with what patients feel has been little opportunity for review. For others, the offer of 'therapy' to 'improve' or 'recover' an individual's pathology and their ability to cope can prove unhelpful and upsetting when it fails to address the broader social circum-stances which fuel the person's underlying distress.

This is certainly not to point a finger of blame at GPs, who in the UK are increasingly working in severely resource-constrained environments with few options to provide other forms of support to those experiencing poverty-related mental distress. Indeed, almost all of the GPs interviewed as part of the DeStress project expressed anger and frustration at the way that they had become caught up in current and previous government drives to cut costs through slashing welfare entitlements and deliver what David Cameron as prime minister called 'a responsible society'. Rather, it is to recognise that while the delivery of widescale mental health treatment must be applauded in circumstances where it genuinely and effectively responds to need, its current entanglement with wider political agendas has resulted in the pathologisation and medicalisation of what are inher-ently social and structural issues, and that this in turn can increase stigma, blame and injustice against those in low-income communities.

At the heart of these issues are questions about where responsibility for health and wellbeing should lie. Governments can facilitate responsibility in citizens when they provide the material and structural resources required for this to become feasible. Yet, within the current neo-liberally oriented era, government and popular rhetoric around individual respons-ibility feed directly into strategies aimed at reducing welfare support, blaming and shaming individuals and communities, and deflecting atten-tion from the responsibilities of those with the power and remit to effect positive change.

Such a situation is clearly inequitable and in fact damaging to people's mental health and wellbeing.

While solutions to this situation ultimately require a fundamental shift in the culture and language of policy and practice, more immediate – and ultimately cost-effective – strategies do exist that may help alleviate, and more effectively respond to, distress within low-income communities. As part of DeStress, we are, for example, working with Health Education England, health practitioners and low-income communities to develop training materials for GPs on how to use the limited time available within consultations to more effectively engage with people experiencing poverty-related distress. A key aspect of this work involves enabling GPs to feel better able to play a supportive and empathic role that encourages patients to reflect on their situation and identify positive ways forward, rather than feeling that they necessarily need to 'fix' patients through diagnosis and treatment.

There is also strong evidence from DeStress that a great deal of distress within low-income communities is caused or exacerbated by social isolation and stigma. Where local community groups (often informal in nature) exist, they have been shown to act as powerful support mechanisms that give people reassurance and a sense of purpose and belonging. Successive UK governments have reduced funding for these activities – yet reinstating and bolstering funding for these kinds of groups would undoubtedly contribute to better wellbeing and more just outcomes.

Acknowledgements

We thank all of the people who gave their time to participate in the DeStress study, as well as the wider DeStress team and advisory board. The DeStress study is funded by the UK Economic and Social Research Council (ref: ES/N018281/1).

Notes

1 The DeStress study took place in two study sites within south-west England.
2 To protect their anonymity, all participant names used in this chapter are pseudonyms.

References

Anderson, S., Brownlie, J. and Given, L., 2009. Therapy Culture? Attitudes towards Emotional Support in Britain. In: A. Park, J. Curtice, K. Thomson, M. Phillips and E. Clery, eds, *British Social Attitudes: The 25th Report*. London: Sage, 155–172.
Ayo, N., 2012. Understanding Health Promotion in a Neoliberal Climate and the Making of Health Conscious Citizens. *Critical Public Health*, 22 (1), 99–105.
Blackburn, D., 2013. *George Osborne's Benefits Speech – Full Text*. Available from: https://blogs.spectator.co.uk/2013/04/george-osbornes-benefits-speech-full-text/ [Accessed 15 April 2018].
Bobek, A., Pembroke, S. and Wickham, J., 2018. *The Social Implications of Precarious Work*. Foundation for European Progressive Studies and Think Tank for Action on Social Change. Available from: www.tasc.ie/download/pdf/living_with_uncertainty_final.pdf [Accessed 23 April 2018].

Busfield, J., 2011. *Mental Illness*. London: Polity.

Clark, D. M., 2011. Implementing NICE Guidelines for the Psychological Treatment of Depression and Anxiety Disorders: The IAPT Experience. *International Review of Psychiatry*, 23 (4), 318–327.

Clement, S., Schauman, O., Graham, T., Maggioni, F., Evans-Lacko, S., Bezborodovs, N., Morgan, C., Rusch, N., Brown, J. S. L. and Thornicroft, G., 2015. What is the Impact of Mental Health-related Stigma on Help-seeking? A Systematic Review of Quantitative and Qualitative Studies. *Psychological Medicine*, 45 (1), 11–27.

Conrad, P., 2007. *The Medicalization of Society: On the Transformation of Human Conditions into Medical Disorders*. Baltimore: John Hopkins University Press.

Crawford, R., 2006. Health as a Meaningful Social Practice. *Health*, 10 (4), 401–420.

Cruickshank, G., MacGillivray, S., Bruce, D., Mather, A., Matthews, K. and Williams, B., 2008. Cross-sectional Survey of Patients in Receipt of Long-term Repeat Prescriptions for Antidepressant Drugs in Primary Care. *Mental Health in Family Medicine*, 5 (2), 105–109.

Davey, C. G. and Chanen, A. M., 2016. The Unfulfilled Promise of the Antidepressant Medications. *Medical Journal of Australia*, 204 (9L), 348–350.

Dowrick, C. and Frances, A., 2013. Medicalising Unhappiness: New Classification of Depression Risks More Patients Being Put on Drug Treatment from which They Will Not Benefit. *British Medical Journal*, 347, f7140.

EXASOL, 2017. *EXASOL Analyzes: Research Shows That Over 64m Prescriptions of Antidepressants are Dispensed Per Year in England. Visualised for the First Time*. EXASOL. Available from: www.exasol.com/en/company/newsroom/news-and-press/2017-04-13-over-64-million-prescriptions-of-antidepressants-dispensed-per-year-in-england/ [Accessed 30 November 2017].

Friedli, L., 2013. 'What We've Tried, Hasn't Worked': The Politics of Assets Based Public Health. *Critical Public Health*, 23 (2), 131–145.

Friedli, L. and Stearn, R., 2015. Positive Affect as Coercive Strategy: Conditionality, Activation and the Role of Psychology in UK Government Workfare Programmes. *Medical Humanities*, 41, 40–47.

Gøtzsche, P. C., 2015. Does Long Term Use of Psychiatric Drugs Cause More Harm Than Good? *British Medical Journal*, 350, h2435.

Harrow, M., Jobe, T. H. and Faull, R. N., 2014. Does Treatment of Schizophrenia with Antipsychotic Medications Eliminate or Reduce Psychosis? A 20-year Multi-follow-up Study. *Psychological Medicine*, 44 (14), 3007–3016.

Kendrick, T., 2015. Long-term Antidepressant Treatment: Time for a Review. *Prescriber*, 26 (19), 7–10.

Kirsch I., Deacon, B. J., Huedo-Medina, T. B., Scoboria, A., Moore, T. J. and Johnson, B. T., 2008. Initial Severity and Antidepressant Benefits: A Meta-analysis of Data Submitted to the Food and Drug Administration. *PLOS Medicine*, 5 (2), e45 doi: 10.1371/journal.pmed.005004.

Leichter, H. M., 1997. Lifestyle Correctness and the New Secular Morality. In: A. M. Brandt and P. Rozin, eds, *Morality and Health*. New York: Routledge, 359–378.

Lewer, D., O'Reilly, C., Mojtabai, R. and Evans-Lacko, S., 2015. Antidepressant Use in 27 European Countries: Associations with Socio-demographic, Cultural and Economic Factors. *British Journal of Psychiatry*, 207 (3), 221–226.

Lupton, D., 1995. *The Imperative of Health: Public Health and the Regulated Body*. London: Sage.

Mojtabai, R. and Olfson, M., 2014. National Trends in Long-term Use of Antidepressant Medications: Results from the U.S. National Health and Nutrition Examination Survey. *Journal of Clinical Psychiatry*, 75 (2), 169–177.

Modini, M., Joyce, S., Myykletun, A., Christensen, H., Bryant, R. A., Mitchell, P. B. and Harvey, S. B., 2016. The Mental Health Benefits of Employment: Results of a Systematic Meta-review. *Australasian Psychiatry*, 24 (4), 331–336.

NatCen, 2013. *Public Attitudes to Poverty and Welfare 1983–2011*. NatCen. Available from: www.natcen.ac.uk/our-research/research/public-attitudes-to-poverty-and-welfare-1983-2011/ [Accessed 3 March 2018].

NHS, 2015. *Improving Access to Psychological Therapies*. NHS. Available from: www.iapt.nhs.uk [Accessed 5 May 2018].

NHS Digital, 2017. Prescriptions Dispensed in the Community, Statistics for England – 2006–2016 [PAS]. NHS. Available from: http://digital.nhs.uk/catalogue/PUB30014 [Accessed 7 June 2018].

Parkin, E. and Powell, T., 2017. *Mental Health Policy in England, Briefing Paper No. CBP 07547*. London: House of Commons Library.

Shaw, I. and Taplin, S., 2007. Happiness and Mental Health Policy: A Sociological Critique. *Journal of Mental Health*, 16 (3), 359–373.

Shildrick, T. and MacDonald, R., 2013. Poverty Talk: How People Experiencing Poverty Deny Their Poverty and Why They Blame 'the Poor'. *Sociological Review*, 61 (2), 285–303.

Tinson, A., Ayrton, C., Barker, K., Born, T. B., Aldridge, H. and Kenway, P., 2016. *Monitoring Poverty and Social Exclusion 2016 (MPSE)*. York: Joseph Rowntree Foundation and New Policy Institute.

Walker, R., 2014. *The Shame of Poverty*. Oxford: Oxford University Press.

WHO, 2017. *Depression and Other Common Mental Disorders: Global Health Estimates*. Geneva: WHO.

Chapter 5

Critical theories of justice and the practice of torture prevention

Danielle Celermajer

Introduction

Questions about the proper relationship between theory and practice have a perennial, as if unresolvable, presence. On the one side, there are politicians seeking 'value for money', practitioners seeking effectiveness, and students seeking the practical relevance of theory. On the other, there are theorists, particularly those whose work is at the more abstract end of the spectrum, who decry the failure of those who make such demands to appreciate the far-reaching, sometimes delayed, impacts of 'good theory'. If transformative theories are to be produced, they need to be afforded intellectual space, unencumbered by instrumentalist demands. A slightly different, but related, response is to defend theory, not on the basis of its distinctive temporality, but rather in terms of the radical nature of the changes it would demand. According to this view, demands made in the name of practice have the perverse effect of rendering relatively superficial any changes that can be proposed. Indeed, for some, such compromise may be precisely what is intended, albeit under the guise of other, nobler motives.

In the field of human rights practice, theory has, traditionally, played a relatively minor or implicit role. Normative and political theories concerning the essential dignity and equality of all persons are what gives shape to the human rights idea, and in turn underpin human rights practice;[1] but such theories are constitutive of the approach rather than providing specific guidance to the practices that fall under its umbrella. Admittedly, there are a few instances where theory has directly engaged with, made demands of, and indeed had an effect on practice. Feminist human rights theories, for example, have illuminated how the human rights canon traditionally assumed and then reified gendered distinctions between the public and private spheres, thereby excluding concern for the violations specifically suffered by women, such as domestic violence or rape in war (Charlesworth *et al.* 1991). These theoretical stances then gave rise to demands that the exclusions generated by this gendered schema be explicitly recognised in human rights law and practice.[2] Moreover, particular theories, such as those concerning the relationship between the media, representations of suffering and human rights (McLagan 2003, Cohen 2013), have influenced the way in which human rights organisations frame and mount campaigns (Gregory 2006).

In recent years, however, one of the oldest theoretical critiques of rights, and almost certainly the oldest from the left, has been rejuvenated with a vengeance.[3] In its original articulation, Marx sought to expose the ideological function that systems that promoted justice through the protection of individual rights, especially in their legal form, played in masking the true causes of injustice and suffering, which were to be found at the level of the structure of economic relations (Marx 1972 [1844]). More recently, and in response to what is seen as an unprecedented ascendency of human rights to the position of the sole remaining authoritative global normative discourse (Moyn 2010), a number of writers have adapted the basic logic of Marx's objection to mount a thoroughgoing critique of the contemporary human rights movement (Klein 2007). As Wendy Brown (2004) puts it, as a 'politics of rhetoric and gesture', human rights 'mislead[s] about the nature of oppressive social forces, and about the scope of the project of transformation required by serious ambitions for justice' (pp. 36–37). Certainly, within this critique of human rights, theorists differ in their approach and emphasis, but they share a common hostility to the level of analysis, or diagnostic frame, that human rights approaches adopt, and claim that human rights approaches pay insufficient attention to the structural underpinnings of injustice.

Pondering what this theoretical analysis might imply for human rights practitioners, one response is that it demands nothing short of abandoning human rights as an approach, at least if they are serious about preventing injustice. The argument here is that at its core, the human rights approach cannot be enhanced to address its problems, because those problems lie with its very logic, or how it understands the nature of injustice. At the extreme, critics accuse human rights not only of failing to address the structural causes of injustice, but of providing ideological cover for those structures and thus enabling their persistence. The obligation to justice would thus entail distancing oneself from such ideological ruses.

Writing human rights approaches off, because of their putative inattention to structure, however, involves three types of errors. The first (empirical) error is conflating into a single characterisation all approaches and projects that adopt the language of human rights, overlooking the range of strategies and politics within what is a broad and internally contested movement. This is evident in, for example, human-rights-based approaches to health, where the distinctive value of human rights includes analysing and attending to the relations of power that create the conditions of ill health (Farmer 2004).

The second (conceptual) error is to assume that human rights approaches have an absolute and unchangeable essence, in this case, one that dooms them to being inimical to structural analyses of injustice. This conceptual essentialism is particularly ironic, given that a number of critical theorists (including Moyn) embrace a genealogical approach, which entails an irreducible indeterminacy with respect to the possibilities of a concept or practice, and a rejection of the view that there exists an ahistorical, essential set of qualities necessarily entailed in any expression of that concept (Golder 2016).

The third error, and one I take up here, concerns a failure to differentiate between the level at which theoretical critique takes place, and the level at which practical interventions occur. For critical theorists, adopting what we might call macro-analytic categories, such as neo-liberalism, cultural imperialism, or patriarchy, may afford access to understanding how persistent and patterned violations are sustained; but it provides little guidance for practitioners, who need to operate at the level of manifest and accessible processes or practices.

For example, in her theoretical work on torture in the context of the Algerian independence movement, Marnia Lazreg drew a powerful and illuminating theoretical link between France's systematic use of torture, and its efforts to fortify imperial power increasingly threatened by an enemy considered to lack the markers of civilisation (Lazreg 2016). While Lazreg's theoretical work can provide political movements thinking through long-term strategies with invaluable insights and assist them in making critical connections, one would be hard pressed to translate her analysis into a prevention strategy for practitioners. This is not to deny the benefit of locating efforts to prevent torture within a broader fight against imperialism, nor the importance of assuming the longer-term project of preventing imperial rule. The specific actions and strategies that comprise any intervention, including the fight against imperialism will however, of necessity, fall short of this 'macro-level' diagnosis or macro-problem. No one simply goes out and 'prevents imperialism', be it political or cultural.

We are thus left with the question, is there a way in which human rights practice can be responsive to theories that illuminate the links between human rights violations and larger structures? The answer that I give in this chapter is, unsurprisingly, yes and no; and yes, only if we differentiate between the levels of critical theory and preventative practice, only if we are prepared to recognise that reform and revolution are not mutually exclusive, and only if we alter what we mean by structure. These qualifications may mean that for the structural thinkers associated with this body of critique, my 'yes' counts as 'no'.

I begin with a brief overview of the structural critique and a discussion of the different demands of theory and practice. I next consider a different group of theories that might also be considered structural, but that do not adopt the type of substructure and superstructure model of neo-Marxist theories. Like neo-Marxist accounts, ecological or systemic theories locate the causes of human rights violations at sites well beyond the dyad of perpetrator and victim, but they offer a far more differentiated and accessible map and guide for intervention. In the final section of the chapter, I consider how, if human rights practice is to be fully informed by ecological and systemic theories, it would benefit from engaging with social theories that help us rethink agency and causality in a less individualistic human-centric manner.

Critical theory and human rights

In recent years, an approach that I will here call neo-Marxist structuralism has gained increasing purchase in the world of human rights scholarship, advocating a strong critical stance towards human rights as an approach to injustice. The most broadly known figure writing in this tradition is the historian Sam Moyn (2010, 2014), but other key theorists include Susan Marks (2011), Naomi Klein (2007), and Wendy Brown (2004). Their basic stance is to admonish human rights approaches for locating their analysis at the level of the individual, thereby obscuring the structural underpinnings of violations, and more specifically in the contemporary context, the rise of neo-liberalism. Nevertheless, they vary in how they understand the politics of the association between human rights and these structural ills. At the extreme, for Brown or Klein for example, human rights and their proponents play an active or at least complicit role in the promotion of neo-liberalism. Others, specifically Moyn, settle for a less accusatory association of temporal coincidence or correlation between the late twentieth-century ascendency of these two phenomena. Theoretically, in the background to these specific objections to human rights lies a more comprehensive social ontology, which posits the actions, as well as the values and ideas, of the individuals who perpetrate or permit and authorise violations as the secondary effects of macro-structural arrangements. Discrete violations are thus but epiphenomena of structural pathologies.

This approach is clearly evident in critical theories on the deployment of international criminal law as a justice intervention in relation to crimes against humanity. Assessing the theories of history and causality assumed in international criminal law, Gerry Simpson argues that 'over-attention to the behaviour of elites or mandarins', combined with an emphasis on legal analyses, 'has resulted in histories that favour a particular genus of human action, namely, the deliberate and premeditated' (Simpson 2014, p. 164). Simpson quotes Richard Evans's succinct portrayal of the distinctive manner in which criminal law must render history, as that of 'morally and politically autonomous individuals, whose decisions reflected in the first place the peculiarities of their own personalities rather than wider forces of any kind' (Evans 2001, p. 161). Or, as Clifford Geertz more wryly put it, 'whatever it is the law is after, it's not the whole story' (Geertz 1983, p. 183).

In its bolder, and perhaps rasher, moments, for example in *The Endtimes of Human Rights* (Hopgood 2013), the indictment is damning. Indeed, a reader who had no direct experience of what human rights practices actually look like (which may be the case for students whose access to the human rights world is entirely academic) could be forgiven for coming to the conclusion that human rights organisations and advocates are variously driven by nefarious motives, complicit with neo-imperial projects, or perhaps simply naïve or stupid. Part of the remit of scholars is certainly to make evident the complex dynamics that are oversimplified in the commonplace morality tales depicting human rights violators and human rights protectors (Mutua 2001). A crude application of a hermeneutics of suspicion (Ricoeur 1970), however, where human rights organisations are exposed as the agents of neo-liberalism or concerned only with their own survival, does little more than flip the script and create another type of morality tale.

As noted earlier, one weakness of much of this literature is its tendency to collapse all human rights practice into a single approach, an error produced, I suspect, by a lack of engagement with what is actually happening in the field, and thus a tendency to think that the human rights movement is reducible to organisations such as Amnesty International, and even then, to their most popular and superficial public representations. This connects with the error discussed above, assuming that there is an essential and unchangeable form and substance to human rights approaches. Thus, an international campaign aimed at punishing the architect of heinous violations is cited as the putative ideal type of the human rights project, which is then assumed to ineluctably give shape to all human rights projects. Any questions about the contingent factors that may have contributed to the particular types of action undertaken by the best-known and most well-funded organisations are ignored.

The next error is quite different, lying not in a misunderstanding of human rights practice or the concept of human rights, but with the nature of critique itself. Here, the failure is to appreciate the level at which critique operates, what can flow from this level of critique, combined with the belief that one can move directly from critique to implications for practice. Critique, in this sense, is quite different from criticism, which responds to a particular object by pointing out what is wrong with it. Critique, by contrast, looks behind or beneath the object, inviting us to become aware of the implicit frames, paradigms, and discursive or organisational schema that make possible the more immediate phenomena that are normally the object of our attention, and that might be the object of criticism. As Judith Butler puts it, 'critique is concerned to identify the conditions of possibility under which a domain of objects appears' (Butler 2009, p. 109). Indeed, when we, or even more so, critiques' authors, look to it to provide practical guidance on immediate problems we, and they, miss its point, which is not to provide answers but to raise questions (Felski 2011). To wield critique as a weapon to accuse practitioners, and implicitly demand that they act otherwise, is thus to misunderstand the nature of the tool and to abuse it. Again, this does not mean that critique should (to paraphrase Marx) remain in the world of theory, and not partake in changing the world (Marx 1972 [1845]).[4] Its role in world-changing is, however, a quite distinctive one that ought not to be confused with direct prescriptions for new forms of practice.[5]

The practical implications of these new critical theoretical engagements with human rights are not direct, clear or distinct; and nor should they be, because those critiques are supposed to act as provocations to reflexivity, including on the conditions, assumptions, and implicit productions of one's own practice. Quick responses would, in this sense, likely do those critiques a disservice, for they demand a much slower form of reflection (Felski 2011). Nevertheless, we might usefully speculate on the types of rethinking and revised practice these critiques of human rights approaches might provoke. For example, in response to Simpson's critique of the indi-vidualising thrust of international criminal law, practitioners might reflect on punishment's expressive function, that is, on the types of stories about wrongdoing that punishment and trials tend to express and thus con-struct. They might then take the trail as an opportunity to provoke conver-sations that go beyond the individualising narrative of guilt or innocence, using other media platforms to explore the broader structural conditions that made the specific abuses possible.

At the same time, the general theoretical insight (that broader struc-tural factors contribute to, or underpin, human rights violations), can be made to do more practical work than this. To do so, however, we need to look beyond macro-critiques, to other theories that come a little closer to the access points for practice, while still carrying the trace of the critical stance. In this regard, I see situational or ecological theories as particularly fertile. These theoretical stances also insist on broadening the lens we bring to diagnosing the causes or conditions of human rights violations, but they do so in a manner that can have direct implications for practice.

Ecological, situational and systems theories

In the aftermath of the Shoah, a pressing dilemma for many people was how so many apparently ordinary people could have participated, more or less directly, in atrocities. To try to make sense of this puzzle, social psychologists intensified their research into obedience and conformity

(Schachter 1959, Kelman 1973). Some of this research, like Asch's (1956) experiments testing what subjects would say when asked to make a very obvious visual judgement after others had made a very obviously incorrect judgement, did not directly bear on questions of violence or violations, but began to fill out the picture of how context and group dynamics shape what hitherto we might have conceptualised as the judgements, choices and free actions of individual agents.

Others, most famously Stanley Milgram in his electric shock experiments (Milgram 1974) and Philip Zimbardo in the Stanford prison experiments (Zimbardo *et al.* 2000), investigated the question of subjects' willingness to commit violent acts by placing randomly selected volunteers in situations where such acts were ordered, authorised, condoned or normalised. Shockingly, both found that people with no particular predisposition towards violence were willing to act with unambiguous cruelty towards strangers. In the case of Milgram's experiments, they did so when an authority figure ordered or instructed them to do so.[6] In the case of Zimbardo's experiments, the young men assigned the role of mock guards were under no direct orders to act in any particular manner, but nevertheless subsequently abused the mock prisoners. These findings shed important light on institutional violence, insofar as the violations seemed to flow from a range of situational factors or cues, such as individuals being placed in positions of unsupervised authority, the wearing of uniforms, the anonymity and staged powerlessness of the victims, and the closed nature of the setting.

Findings from these experiments provided a rejoinder to dispositional theories of violence, which located the principal causes at the level of the individuals who order or commit wrongful acts. By contrast, situational theories located the principal causal or conditioning factors in the situation or context within which agents were located. Importantly, the more sophisticated theoretical models that emerged from this work did not adopt a crude structuralism, whereby individual actions might be cast as the mere effects of structural causes. Rather, human agency was itself recast as radically situated.

Milgram and Zimbardo's work drew attention to a particular set of situational and systemic factors, those in the immediate organisational environment, but it pointed more broadly to a general theoretical frame that understood actions and individual value orientations or judgements as embedded in broader systems. These might be placed under a broad umbrella of systems or ecological theories. Uri Bronhoffer's ecological systems model, for example, as illustrated in Figure 5.1, understands individual behaviour as influenced by a range of systems, from the most immediate to the apparently more remote. Developed originally to understand child development, the theory can be applied to understand the actions of any individual or group of people. Representations of the model, both pictorial and in our imagination, tend to map the different systems in a fairly linear, two-dimensional and hierarchical manner. A more accurate way to imagine these systems would be as only partially independent fields within a multi-dimensional space, organised by relative differences in density, internal rules and dynamics, which nevertheless fold into each other and are co-constitutive.

Like structural critiques, such theories insist on the error involved in abstracting a particular violation, and the individuals involved in it, from the larger systems of which they are a part. At the same time, for our purposes, they differ from macro-structural theories in important respects. First, they are not a priori committed to the primacy of any particular system or any one part of the overall field. Indeed, here it is not simply a matter of rejecting the idea that we can know beforehand whether economic structures, the form of law, cultural factors, or political-level factors are the most important, or ultimate, causes. Rather, by mapping these different systems as a multi-dimensional space, it is possible to recognise a fluidity in causal ordering, and the co-constitutional relations between systems and structures. Moreover, because their model of causality is systemic or ecological and not linear, they avoid the danger of reductive

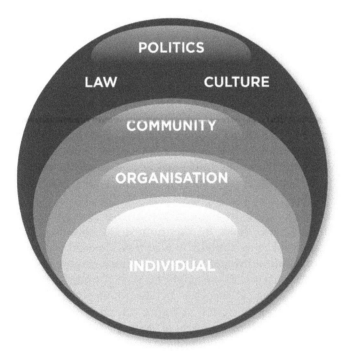

Figure 5.1 Bronfenbrenner's ecological systems model.

or final causal stories or, to put it differently, of abstracting what is located as a cause or conditioning factor from its own causes or conditioning factors. To take the example of the Stanford prison experiment, one can identify the closed prison environment and the absence of clear rules regulating the behaviour of guards as factors that conditioned the use of violence by the 'guards', at the same time as recognising that prison environments and rules over guards are themselves shaped within larger legal, political and cultural systems. Where one ought to intervene with a view to shifting the overall systemic dynamics is not in itself given by the theory, and so cannot be determined in advance. The theory thus provides an orientation, but not a predetermined answer.

Moreover, unlike macro-theories, which insist that we need to attend to macro-patterns or structures (such as neo-liberalism) if we are to understand the aetiology of specific violations, these theoretical approaches map and thus encourage us to attend to the specific institutional settings, practices and processes that generate the violation. In some cases, systems, processes or practices may be fairly proximate to the violation, but in others, they are more indirectly or remotely connected. Similarly, in some cases the factors may be fairly abstract (such as discriminatory attitudes to certain groups), and in other cases they are quite concrete (such as the absence of proximate sanctions for infractions of an abstract rule or formal law).

The practice of torture prevention

A recent project seeking to develop more effective approaches to preventing torture in the police in Nepal and Sri Lanka (Celermajer 2015, 2018) illustrates how this theoretical frame might be taken up in human rights practice. This project was specifically concerned not with the spectacular torture that most often attracts public attention, but with the everyday and systematic forms of torture inflicted as a matter of routine throughout these institutions. Consistent with the need to ground prevention practices in an empirically informed theory of change (Nation *et al.* 2003), our team commenced by trying to build a rich understanding of the causal or contributing factors underpinning torture. Informed by a systemic theoretical framework, we recognised the need to cast our research net broadly. As it transpired, our research revealed an enormous range of factors operating across different spheres: in politics; in the criminal justice system; in the legal system; in the broader society or culture; in discourses and ideologies; as well as at the level of security-sector organisations themselves, and at the level of the individual personnel. They included factors such as political interference in the work of law enforcement agencies; clientism and cronyism, whereby local political leaders used the police to prosecute their partisan interests; social norms concerning righteous violence against so-called delinquent individuals such as drug addicts; the admission by courts of evidence obtained under torture; the unwillingness of allied professionals such as doctors to document torture when they suspect it has occurred; the fact that local police stations need to meet quotas of charges laid if they are to receive resources; intra-organisational violence; boredom and isolation of security-sector personnel; and the lack of investigative skills amongst frontline police personnel (Grewal and Celermajer 2015a, 2015b).

A systems or ecological theoretical frame allowed us to map these different types of factors, and to think through how they shaped both each other and practices of law enforcement. For example, in Sri Lanka, we found general societal approval of the use of 'corrective violence' against certain types of people, specifically those considered to be lacking the markers of 'civilised' subjects. We also found a legal and political system that failed to hold police personnel to account where they violated human rights norms or laws, and an organisational context in which there were numerous demand-side factors on police personnel to get confessions and display toughness against criminals. These both reinforced each other and fed into a generalised expectation amongst police that violence against certain classes of people was unproblematic, if not expected (Munasinghe and Celermajer 2017).

From this example, one can see how ecological system theories can equip practitioners in a number of ways. Most obviously, they suggest that to be effective, interventions need to be multi-systemic, addressing the different parts of the system that contribute to, or sustain, the particular problem being targeted. This may seem obvious, but the field of torture prevention is replete with one-dimensional projects that operate in isolation from the broader conditions that sustain the problem that their discrete intervention is targeting. Training police in human rights norms, for example, and more specifically teaching them that the use of violence to obtain confessions is morally and legally impermissible, is unlikely to have much impact if police officers continue to be subject to higher-order demands to produce evidence. Nor will banning the use of torture to obtain confessions help where police are not equipped, resourced or skilled to achieve the outcomes they are pressured to produce in ways that respect human rights. Similarly, mandating medical inspections will be of little use, without also ensuring the availability of properly trained medical practitioners, attending to the conditions that have to be met if they are going to be able to operate independently, and creating reforms within the broader criminal justice and judicial system to ensure that their reports carry authority. Hypothetically, one could work this out without having an ecological map, but having one is helpful in plotting the different factors that feed into, and sustain, the focused upon problem.

Ecological system theories can also assist practitioners by helping to map how the different spheres or institutions within the overall system shape each other and how they are located vis-à-vis each other in a broader field of power. This in turn can provide guidance for working out where in the overall multi-systematic field the most effective intervention points will be. Given how frequently the choice about what type of intervention to pursue is given by the habitual practices of organisations, or assumptions about what is effective, this type of strategic mapping can make a significant contribution to effectiveness. As Carver and Handley document, for example, there is a significant gap between the impact that formal legal regulations requiring certain preventive measures have, and the substantive implementation of those measures (Carver and Handley 2016, p. 52), and yet, advocating legal reform is often a default strategy for human rights organisations.

In the case of the torture prevention project that we conducted, we learned this lesson the hard way. From the outset, we had specified that our intervention was to take place at the level of security-sector organisations. But when we mapped our empirical findings using an ecological systems model, it became clear that in Sri Lanka especially, security-sector organisations were, to a significant extent, subordinate to political actors. Because of this, unless we were also able to intervene at the political level, our ability to affect any type of change in security organisations would be highly constrained. At the same time, any changes that security-sector personnel made or tried to make would be stymied by the operation of factors at the political level. By contrast, in Nepal, where we also conducted work, the organisational level had significant autonomy, and as such operating at this level alone was potentially sufficient to alter certain structures and processes that contributed to torture.

Finally, and this links back to the need to navigate a path between system and agent, ecological theories suggest that to effectively prevent torture, the focus should be on altering the situations or contexts in which individuals judge and act, by, for example, altering the conditions of detention. We now have good empirical support for this hypothesis. A recent analysis of the impact of different torture prevention strategies across 26 countries (Carver and Handley 2016) indicated that the most effective interventions were those that brought about changes in the conditions of detention and the organisational environment within which security-sector personnel acted. Ending impunity by punishing individual perpetrators *does* contribute to the reduction of torture, but to a lesser extent.

Systemic or ecological theories thus usefully draw practitioners' attention away from the immediate site of perpetration or violation to the background conditions that render violations possible and sustain them. They do not, however, of themselves, provide the theoretical resources for making sense of the tensions between agent responsibility and systemic conditioning that inevitably come with them, and we are likely to be left with the persistent intuition that human agents are the cause of wrongs such as torture. Such theoretical aporias do not in themselves impede practitioners from working directly on the systems in which agents are embedded. The persistence of our moral intuitions, however, and the feelings of blame and anger that they entail, may make it difficult for practitioners to make a convincing case for more systemic approaches.

Some new theoretical resources for rethinking agency

Over the last 20 years, theorists have articulated a number of frameworks to take us beyond the agent–structure problems generated in classical social theory. In this regard, actor–network theories, assemblage theories, new materialisms and post-humanisms, though importantly different, share some important features. They insist that one cannot coherently abstract any particular social phenomenon, including an unjust act or system, and then explain its aetiology using a linear causal narrative, especially one that places human agency at the centre. Rather, any particular phenomenon is embedded in a complex of factors that stand in relations of interdependence or mutual arising.

This complex of factors includes not only individual people, collectives, structures such as economic relations and discourses, but also the more-than-human world – the arrangement of buildings, technological systems, material resources and so on. In this respect, factors that have traditionally been cast as objects whose contribution is limited to how they are manipulated by humans, are reinvested with a type of agency, although in all of these accounts, agency needs to be radically reimagined as distributed, dispersed or networked. Here, I note three theoretical claims that can supplement the mapping that ecological theories produce by helping us rethink the type of causal story we need to tell about how individual human agents and systems 'fit' to produce violations.

First, they assume flat ontologies, so that no particular type of entity or institution is *prima facie* causally privileged, and their relative location in the overall field of power is fluid. We can see this clearly for example in the work of critical human geographers, who reject the notion or model of scale in favour of the notion of site, where site is understood, as Sallie Marston and her co-authors put it, as 'an emergent property of its interacting human and non-human inhabitants'. Such a site ontology, they argue, 'provides the explanatory power' to account for the ways that objects, such as the built environment, for example, 'come to function as an ordering force in relation to the practices of humans arranged in conjunction with it' (Marston *et al.* 2005, p. 425).

Beyond helping us rethink the dynamic of systems, this approach is particularly useful because it does not assume, and therefore commit us to, a fixed set of sub-systems – politics, law, the economy, society and so on. Nor does it assume that these stand in particular types of relationship or that they are organised in a static way. This allows for a more open-ended appreciation of the ways in which those fields may in fact be constituted in different social and political contexts, and an aliveness to the ways in which they shift. The scalar imagination that has been so prevalent, albeit implicitly, in most structural or systems theories gives way here to a far more fluid approach.

Recognising this fluidity or instability becomes particularly important as one moves between contexts. In her ethnographic research on police encounter killings in India, for example, Beatrice Jauregui (2016) shows how in the Indian post-colonial context, the police occupy a highly unstable position in a field where multiple actors are in a constant contest for power and authority, the police being just one amongst them, and with no protected privilege. Here, assumptions that we are likely to bring about the meaning or operation of law based on the field of power in liberal democracies may impede our ability to properly map the field of power that is actually at play.

Second, as I already noted, these approaches radicalise what we mean by agency. They do not simply embed human agency, but decentre it altogether. William Connolly writes, for example, that once we 'come to terms with a cosmos composed of interacting force-fields invested with differing speeds and degrees of agency', any particular zone of study 'needs to have both a microscopic and a planetary dimension folded into it, with the relevant features shifting, depending on the problem complex under scrutiny' (Connolly 2013, p. 401). This type of decentred conception of agency remains counter-intuitive for most of us; nevertheless, it opens the possibility of a much better way for thinking about causality than a framework that still assumes as basic ontological categories the terms structure, system and agent.

Third, and perhaps most radically, these theories see systems as self-organising, or 'onto-genetic'. Again, as Marston puts it, 'the dynamic properties of matter produce a multiplicity of complex relations and singularities that sometimes lead to the creation of new, unique events and entities, but more often to relatively redundant orders and practices' (Marston *et al.* 2005, p. 422). On the one hand, this notion of onto-genetic systems presents a real challenge in imagining what it would even mean to intervene.[7] This dilemma deepens once one realises that there is no outside to the system, and so no privileged place from which one could look into the system and intervene.[8] Perhaps, though, taking the transcendence out of intervention would not be a bad thing. Recognising that there is no outside of the system from which to intervene might itself usefully illuminate the ways in which human rights organisations and practices are themselves also implicated in broader dynamics.

To illustrate, a leader from one of the principal human rights organisations in Israel recently described for me why they had decided to no longer mount legal challenges against laws passed by the Knesset or against alleged violations committed by the Israel Defence Forces. Over the years, he explained, it became clearer to them that, although his organisation saw itself as outside the system, it was in fact part of that system. This was evident for example in the way that the Israeli Government cited NGO activities as evidence of the vibrancy of liberal democracy, freedom of speech and a culture of respect for human rights in Israel. This recognition obviously poses challenges for what to do next, but if the analysis is correct, doing more of the same is unlikely to be productive in achieving the objective of preventing human rights violations. Presumably what is required is an intervention that includes oneself as an object in the analysis.

Concluding thoughts

Particularly in the face of injustices and violations as heinous and trenchant as torture, there is a danger that people committed to change will look to others' approaches – in the realms of theory or practice – and fault them, in one way or other, for missing the point. No doubt, some theories and some practices get it wrong in their analysis of the problem, or their understanding of how to bring about change. In some instances, though, the faults that they see in each other are artefacts of the type of work that theory and practice do, and sometimes these are profoundly different.

Nevertheless, even theories that may seem relatively abstract, and ones that afford new ontological schemas for thinking about causality, can offer resources for practitioners, especially those who want to critically reflect upon how they go about their work, or who are looking for new frames to make sense of problems and imagine solutions. The work of translation across those spheres requires patience, permeability and a recognition that although we seem to be approaching a common problem, the world 'opens to us', as Arendt wrote, from distinctive and often very different perspectives (Arendt 2005, pp. 14–18). As she insisted, however, our care for the world, and the creation of a common world, requires our recognising the truth in each perspective.

Notes

1 See for example Griffin (2008).
2 Framed thus, it would appear that theory precedes practice, although in areas such as feminism, it is clear that social movements, a form of practice, also inform theory. See Stammers (2009).

3 The oldest being the conservative criticism originally articulated by Burke, who faulted rights for being abstract, meaning they had no foundation in reality (Burke 1999). My interest here is on progressive rather than conservative theoretical criticisms.
4 The reference is to Thesis 11, 'The philosophers have only interpreted the world in various ways; the point, however, is to *change* it.'
5 In this regard, Marx's Thesis 11 has also been misread. It was not, as Cornel West argues, a 'call to blind activism', but an insistence that all theory also recognise itself as 'under-a-description' (West 1991, pp. 67–68).
6 Importantly, Milgram included a number of experimental variants thereby showing that factors such as the perceived authority and gender of the figure giving the orders, the way that the acts or the victims are described, the proximity to the victim, and the presence of dissenting subjects have significant impacts on levels of obedience.
7 I leave to the side here difficult questions about responsibility raised by actor–network theory.
8 It's worth noting that this problem is not new. One can already see its contours in Spinoza's critique in *The Ethics* (Spinoza 1994) of the notion of a providential God who causes things to happen, and with that, our picture of ourselves as little gods capable of manipulating the world, including other people, to achieve an abstract moral end we have defined as good. If there is only one substance, with infinite modes that are arranged in necessary causal relations, one part cannot decide – from a position of assumed transcendence – to change the others because this part, or person, deems that other parts, persons or actions are violating fundamental norms.

References

Arendt, H., 2005. *The Promise of Politics*. New York: Schocken Books.
Asch, S. E., 1956. Studies of Independence and Conformity: I. A Minority of One against a Unanimous Majority. *Psychological Monographs: General and Applied*, 70 (9), 1–70.
Brown, W., 2004. 'The Most We Can Hope For…': Human Rights and the Politics of Fatalism. *South Atlantic Quarterly*, 103 (2), 451–463.
Burke, E., 1999. *Reflections on the Revolution in France*. Oxford: Oxford University Press.
Butler, J., 2009. The Sensibility of Critique: Response to Asad and Mahmood. In: T. Asad, W. Brown, J. Butler and S. Mahmood, eds, *Is Critique Secular? Blasphemy, Injury, and Free Speech*. Berkeley: Townsend Center for the Humanities, 101–136.
Carver, R. and Handley, L., 2016. *Does Torture Prevention Work?* Liverpool: Liverpool University Press.
Celermajer, D., 2015. *Project Overview: Enhancing Human Rights Protections in the Security Sector in the Asia Pacific Project*. Sydney: University of Sydney.
Celermajer, D., 2018. *The Prevention of Torture: An Ecological Approach*. New York: Cambridge University Press.
Charlesworth, H., Chinkin, C. and Wright, S., 1991. Feminist Approaches to International Law. *American Journal of International Law*, 85 (4), 613–645.
Cohen, S., 2013. *States of Denial: Knowing about Atrocities and Suffering*. Cambridge: Polity Press.

Connolly, W. E., 2013. The 'New Materialism' and the Fragility of Things. *Millennium*, 41 (3), 399–412.

Evans, R. J., 2001. *In Defence of History*. London: Granta Books.

Farmer, P., 2004. *Pathologies of Power: Health, Human Rights, and the New War on the Poor*. Berkeley and Los Angeles: University of California Press.

Felski, R., 2011. Critique and the Hermeneutics of Suspicion. *M/C Journal*, 15 (1).

Geertz, C., 1983. *Local Knowledge: Further Essays in Interpretative Anthropology*. New York: Basic Books.

Golder, B., 2016. On the Genealogy of Human Rights: An Essay on (Nostalgia) Nostaligia. *Australian Journal of Human Rights*, 22 (1), 17–36.

Gregory, S., 2006. Transnational Storytelling: Human Rights, WITNESS, and Video Advocacy. *American Anthropologist*, 108 (1), 195–204.

Grewal, K. and Celermajer, D., 2015a. *EHRP Issues Paper 3: Human Rights in the Sri Lankan Law Enforcement and Security Sector*. Sydney: University of Sydney.

Grewal, K, and Celermajer, D., 2015b. *EHRP Issues Paper 4: Human Rights in the Nepali Law Enforcement and Security Sector*. Sydney: University of Sydney.

Griffin, J., 2008. *On Human Rights*. Oxford: Oxford University Press.

Hopgood, S., 2013. *The Endtimes of Human Rights*. Ithaca, NY: Cornell University Press.

Jauregui, B. A., 2016. *Provisional Authority: Police, Order, and Security in India*. Chicago: University of Chicago Press.

Kelman, H. C., 1973. Violence without Moral Restraint: Reflections on the Dehumanization of Victims and Victimizers. *Journal of Social Issues*, 29 (4), 25–61.

Klein, N., 2007. *The Shock Doctrine: The Rise of Disaster Capitalism*. London: Penguin.

Lazreg, M., 2016. *Torture and the Twilight of Empire: From Algiers to Baghdad*. Princeton: Princeton University Press.

Marks, S., 2011. Human Rights and Root Causes. *Modern Law Review*, 74 (1), 57–78.

Marston, S. A., Jones, J. P. and Woodward, K., 2005. Human Geography without Scale. *Transactions of the Institute of British Geographers*, 30 (4), 416–432.

Marx, K., 1972 [1844]. On the Jewish Question. In: R. C. Tucker, ed., *The Marx-Engels Reader*. New York: Norton, 26–46.

Marx, K., 1972 [1845]. Theses on Feuerbach. In: R. C. Tucker, ed., *The Marx-Engels Reader*. New York: Norton, 143–145.

McLagan, M., 2003. Principles, Publicity, and Politics: Notes on Human Rights Media. *American Anthropologist*, 105 (3), 605–612.

Milgram, S., 1974. *Obedience to Authority: An Experimental View*. New York: Harper & Row.

Moyn, S., 2010. *The Last Utopia*. Cambridge, MA: Harvard University Press.

Moyn, S., 2014. The Future of Human Rights. *Sur: International Journal of Human Rights*, 11 (20), 57–66.

Munasinghe, V. and Celermajer, D., 2017. Acute and Everyday Violence in Sri Lanka. *Journal of Contemporary Asia*, 47 (4), 615–640.

Mutua, M. W., 2001. Savages, Victims, and Saviors: The Metaphor of Human Rights. *Harvard International Law Journal*, 42 (1), 201–245.

Nation, M., Crusto, C., Wandersman, A., Kumpfer, K. L., Seybolt, D., Morrisey-Kane, E. and Davino, K., 2003. What Works in Prevention: Principles of Effective Prevention Programs. *American Psychologist*, 58 (6–7), 449–456.

Ricoeur, P., 1970. *Freud and Philosophy: An Essay on Interpretation.* Trans. D. Savage. New Haven, CT: Yale University Press.

Schachter, S., 1959. *The Psychology of Affiliation.* Stanford, CA: Standford University Press.

Simpson, G., 2014. Linear Law: The History of International Criminal Law. In: C. Schwobel, ed., *Critical Approaches to International Law.* Oxford and New York: Routledge, 159–179.

Spinoza, B., 1994. *A Spinoza Reader: The Ethics and Other Works.* Trans. E. Curley. Princeton: Princeton University Press.

Stammers, N., 2009. *Human Rights and Social Movements.* Chicago: University of Chicago Press.

West, C., 1991. *The Ethical Dimensions of Marxist Thought.* New York: New York University Press.

Zimbardo, P. G., Maslach, C. and Haney, C., 2000. Reflections on the Stanford Prison Experiment: Genesis, Transformations, Consequences. In: T. Blass, ed., *Obedience to Authority: Current Perspectives on the Milgram Paradigm.* Mahwah, NJ: Lawrence Erlbaum, 193–237.

Chapter 6

Poverty in rich countries

Damage, difference and possibilities for justice

kylie valentine

What is the nature of poverty in rich countries? One representation is in terms of income inequality, which is usually built from population-level data such as income surveys and tax records (Gornick and Jäntti 2014, Piketty 2014). Another is of material and social deprivation, or the things that people do not have and cannot do, because they cannot afford them (Lansley and Mack 2015, Saunders 2015). A third is of depleted health and life expectancy, of lives lived with huge disparities in chronic disease and injury (Murray *et al.* 2006). Each of these accounts is important, because it focuses attention on the seriousness and scope of inequality and disadvantage as a policy problem. Other representations of poverty are more concerned with how it is lived, experienced and perpetuated. They build on the methodological practices of ethnography (Edin and Shaefer 2015, Desmond 2016) and its epistemological field of cultural production (Bourgois 1995, Bourdieu 1999). They deploy oral histories and labour histories and tell the stories of neighbourhoods (Peel 2003). These are also important: not because they tell the 'real' story – all stories are mediated – but because they focus attention on the everyday experiences of poverty, on the circumstances that produce it and the people produced by it.

These latter representations of poverty, which recount its lived experience, are familiar in policy and media as well as scholarship, and are laden with accounts of agency, choice and behaviour. Poverty operates in the international and institutional domains, but is also embodied, domestic and intimate. Since poverty was first studied in rich cities, the everyday choices of the poor – the food eaten, the cultural products consumed and the languages spoken – have been subject to criticism and derision (Jones 2013). These days, nominal equality of access to education and employment is claimed as proof that the acquisition of resources is available to everyone. Inequalities in health, education and employment are treated as moral questions for which individual people can be blamed. Chronic disease is strongly associated with poverty, and the diet and exercise practices of the poor are roundly castigated. When school systems cannot support the social and educational needs of children from poor house-holds, their parents are frequently sanctioned and blamed. The routine labelling of the unemployed as 'bludgers' finds its way into policy settings, where the unemployed are surveilled, immiserised and stigmatised.

All of this is contested, of course. Advocacy and scholarship point to the constraints on the choices faced by the poor, and the impact of ongoing deprivation on health, wellbeing and capacity to perform in competitive educational and employment settings. Differences in the everyday worlds of the poor and the privileged are analysed in terms of habitus and may be defended as class cultures (Haylett 2003, Skeggs 2011). Social practices which are universally accepted as malign, most notably child maltreatment and family violence, are contextualised in terms of intergenerational deprivation and social determinants (Bourgois 1995).

Discussion around poverty may start, in other words, with tidy charts or coefficients, but when concerned with the lives of the poor, the discussion becomes distinctly messy. This chapter is concerned with those who are depicted in 'poverty porn' television shows as chaotic and combative, and often described in policy terms as 'deeply excluded' or 'multiply disadvan-taged'. Considering the question of justice for these groups is a key task in addressing the messiness of poverty.

This is not to say that there is a homogeneous character to poverty, or that its most pernicious manifestations are experienced by everyone who is poor. It is possible to write about poverty by honouring the dignity of the (very many) people who do not maltreat their children or gamble or use alcohol or other drugs problematically, who manage to pay their rent on time and seek help when it is needed – and a rich history of scholarship has done exactly this (Fine 1995, Swadener and Lubeck 1995). Yet when everyday life is impacted upon by policy, through welfare quarantining, drug testing and the practices of child protection agencies, and when the effects of poverty are discernible in everyday miseries and suffering, to neglect those who *do* seem to act against their own best interests seems a dodge of the critical questions of poverty and justice.

To be clear, the figure of the undeserving poor person, resistant to change, making choices that condemn them to stagnation, is a mythic figure, an easy target for policy and public opprobrium but a drastically simplified caricature. The critical response to the deployment of this figure has been, and should be, to question the empirical accuracy of its figuring of poverty and to explain the social determinants of everyday behaviour. Yet, as Shildrick and colleagues argue (2016), the usual critical response also contains the caveat that there *is* a lived experience of poverty that resembles the caricature: the caveat says that these 'troubled' or 'multiproblem' people represent a 'small group' (Shildrick *et al.* 2016). The size of this group is not my concern here. As I have argued elsewhere (valentine 2015), we do not know how many there are. Regardless of the number, the impact of this type of poverty is significant – disproportion-ately on Indigenous people and communities. Services designed for them do not work as intended because of their failure to 'engage' with support, with unerring regularity and at significant cost. Children are removed from families and placed in out-of-home care, families are made homeless, people are released from prison only to die from drug overdoses or return again to custody. The most marginalised – the parents of children in out-of-home care, those who experience the compounded disadvantages of the criminal justice system – are those whose disadvantage is compounded by social stigma and opprobrium.

To begin, I will consider the ways in which questions of agency and choice have been treated in poverty scholarship, and how they are engaged with in Nancy Fraser's influential theory of justice. My aim is to argue that theoretically rich and subtle *analyses* of agency may not be suffi-cient for *normative* claims to justice. Moreover, when agency is incorpor-ated into normative claims, it is increasingly described in terms of difference and damage, and calls to justice are based on reparation for harm. I conclude by proposing some alternatives to this construction of poverty-as-difference-as-damage, drawing on recent feminist legal and Indigenous scholarship.

Explaining poverty: agency and structure

Poverty scholarship is distributed and multidisciplinary. However, it is pos-sible to categorise analyses of poverty's causes, and of where policy inter-ventions should be targeted, as pivoting on the distinction between individual agency and social structure. Broadly speaking, 'agency'-based accounts focus on the choices and behaviours of poor people, while 'struc-ture'-based accounts focus on the role played by social systems and institu-tions in creating and reproducing economic and social inequalities.

A notorious recent example of the former is the underclass thesis. After visiting Britain in 1989, political scientist Charles Murray argued for the existence of an underclass there which was characterised by 'illegitimacy, crime and drop-out from the labour force' (cited in Levitas 1998, p. 17). More recently, he has made the same diagnosis for the USA itself (Murray 2013), arguing that some sections of society have lost the 'founding virtues' of honesty, industriousness, marriage, and religion. Essentially, the underclass offers a culturalist explanation for the intractability of poverty and its effects. According to Murray, and other writers such as Lawrence Mead (2013) who have advanced similar accounts, social security policies have eroded families and communities by making it too easy for lone mothers to raise children and creating pathological communities in which children are inadequately socialised and the value of hard work eroded (cited in Levitas 1998, p. 17).

More recently, the neurobiologist Adam Perkins claims to have diagnosed a 'welfare trait' in the poor, which is also the fault of the welfare state. In Perkins's formulation, the welfare state 'erodes human capital by encouraging the proliferation of an "employment-resistant personality profile"' (cited in Meloni 2016, para. 6). These antisocial, rule-breaking and irresponsible people not only 'suffer impaired life outcomes, but also transmit that difficulty to their children and thus risk damaging the life chances of the next generation' (cited in Meloni 2016, para. 6). Murray and Mead write of values, Perkins of epigenetic plasticity, but all contribute to a long tradition. As Michael Katz writes (2013, p. ix), the idea that 'some poor people are undeserving of help because they brought their poverty on themselves' is an enduring theme in the policy response to poverty.

Murray and Perkins focus on the behaviours of the poor, but their arguments are directed at governments. In contrast, more structurally informed accounts are also directed at the state, but rather than arguing that the state is to blame for creating dysfunctional individuals, they point to the systems and institutional practices that perpetuate poverty and disadvantage. A long tradition of scholarship on the welfare state has concentrated on questions of equity and distribution, and the responsibilities of governments in ensuring social protection (summarised in Deacon 2004, Welshman 2004). Broadly speaking, writers within this tradition are concerned far less with the behaviour of the poor than with the responsibilities of governments (although, as Welshman (2004) argues, this characterisation is a simplification). It has been argued that scholars such as Richard Titmuss and John Kenneth Galbraith, whose writing is so central to this tradition, neglected the questions of agency and behaviour, and this was in part responsible for the emergence of the more conservative individualistic accounts of poverty offered by writers such as Murray and Perkins (Deacon 2004, Welshman 2004, p. 226).

Historically, then, agency-based accounts have tended to be politically conservative: hostile to the welfare state, individualising and inclined to treat everyday cultures and practices as symptoms of social decline. In contrast, more structural accounts have tended to be politically progressive: indebted in broad terms to socialist history and theory, concerned with the responsibility of the state as a redistributive agent, and interested in the sociological and political meanings of everyday cultures and practices.

In recent years, however, the distinction between conservative agency-based accounts and progressive structural accounts (always a simplification) has broken down. The works of influential theorists such as Foucault and Giddens have been used to study 'welfare subjects' as reflexive and agential, acting with autonomy and choice within social structures and both formed by and acting on these structures (Williams and Popay 1999). Scholars of working-class cultures argue that representations of the

undeserving poor exemplify their figuring as antithetical to the contemporary reflexive citizen: they are represented as 'abject and irresponsible, ungovernable, dirty white, pointless and useless, supposedly refusing
not only to accrue value to themselves, but also represented as a drain on
the nation and a blockage to the development of cosmopolitan modernity
of others' (Skeggs 2011, pp. 502–503). Many structural accounts of
poverty, with their calls for social intervention and redistribution, are also
characterised by concerns more closely associated with agency-based
accounts, notably a focus on the dispositions and behaviours of the poor
as necessary targets for intervention (valentine 2015).

Theorising justice and poverty: recognition, respect, rationality

So far, I have considered how the everyday lives and practices of the poor
are often understood within the academic and policy literatures. How are
these lives and practices figured in accounts of poverty that are not only
analytic, but normative? How, in other words, do they figure in accounts
of justice?

Most accounts of poverty and disadvantage, whether based on agency
or structure, are normative in some way. Murray and Perkins, and others
concerned with the underclass thesis, imply what *should* happen, in addition to diagnosing, in Malthusian fashion, what apparently is happening.
Those writing in the social democratic tradition of Titmuss advocate more
explicitly for fairness and equality. Most of the better-known accounts of
poverty do not, however, advance a formal theory of justice. Nancy Fraser
is among those who do, and hers is the most influential in social policy
research. Fraser's work is multi-dimensional and nuanced, but has
changed over the two decades since it was first introduced, especially in
her development of recognition theory in collaboration with Axel
Honneth (Fraser and Honneth 2003). Nevertheless, its core arguments
remain intact: namely, that injustice operates in the economic, cultural/
symbolic and representational spheres, and that justice can only be
achieved if redress is made in each of these spheres. Economic injustice
can manifest in the exploitation of labour, poorly paid or unsafe work, or
material deprivation. Symbolic injustice manifests in cultural domination,
being misrecognised or rendered invisible, or being disparaged and
stereotyped (Fraser 1995). Access to the arenas in which claims for justice
can be made are also critical, so redistribution (economic justice) and
recognition (cultural justice) must also be related to representation
(Fraser *et al.* 2004).

Just as the distinction between 'agency' and 'structure' creates an arti-
ficial separation between mutually constitutive phenomena, Fraser's distinction between the 'economic' and 'cultural' realms has been criticised

by Judith Butler as neglecting the interdependence of these realms (Butler 1998). Notwithstanding this, Fraser's conceptualisation remains useful, as does the distinction between agency and structure, because it identifies the harms that disadvantage brings to bear on people. Even if disrespect and deprivation are mutually intertwined, they can be felt, measured and addressed in different ways. Just as importantly, even if they are mutually reinforcing, they may have independent effects and manifestations, and interventions to address any one of them will not necessarily address the others. The lessons from Fraser in practical and policy terms is that disadvantage has economic and social dimensions, which means in turn that interventions to address disadvantage need to have economic and social objectives.

However, while Fraser is concerned about the harms done to the poor at the level of everyday practice – harms to do with language, stigma, stereotyping and devaluation – she is magisterially unconcerned with the everyday practices of the poor themselves. Sociological debates about the agency and choices associated with disadvantage have little place in her work, because agency is not necessary to her conceptualisation. Unlike Rawls's theory of justice, which views citizens as reasonable and rational (Rawls 1958), Fraser makes no claims about the rationality of people, only to that which is owed to them. Although she takes issue with a Habermasian public sphere of deliberative democracy in which social status distinctions are bracketed off (Habermas 1989 [1962]), arguing that what she calls 'subaltern counterpublics' will always be disadvantaged in unequal societies, she says nothing specifically about how these distinctions are made manifest (Fraser 1997). Fraser deploys a historically informed socialist optimism about the capacity of the poor and a trenchant analysis of the material and discursive injustices wrought upon the poor, but engages barely at all with the ways in which poverty is experienced and lived. Rationality and agency are such fraught concepts in social policy research that their absence from Fraser's work may be one reason for its influence: it provides a model for discussing justice for the poor while circumventing the need to discuss how the poor behave.

Yet there are costs to this influence. More specifically, there are negative consequences attendant to Fraser's theory of justice being so unconcerned with everyday practice, while other narratives around policy are so concerned with it. First, as noted earlier, when everyday practices and behaviours are argued to be the cause of poverty, as conservative scholars and politicians do, any account of justice needs to incorporate the people whose behaviours are so problematised. Claims for justice for the 'deserving' poor are challenging in settings where poverty is maligned, but even more difficult to advance for those judged not to be deserving. Second, sociological analyses of why people appear to act against their best interests are useful, but do not necessarily advance any normative claims.

Third, while Fraser's remains a highly influential theory of justice, justice is also called for in practical ways, in policy and advocacy, and in guide-books and training for social workers and human services. But, as I argue below, the bases of some of these calls for practical justice may be less useful and riskier than they seem.

Claiming practical justice: trauma and damage

A strong and growing demand is for practical justice as redress for the harms and trauma which have created people who are damaged. The organising principle within this argument is that significant trauma in childhood has lifelong effects on mental health and functioning, includ-ing poor outcomes in school, impaired development, psychiatric distress, family violence, child abuse and neglect, and alcohol and other drugs misuse. Put another way, the suggestion here is that manifestations of poverty are manifestations of trauma, and that justice is a question of redressing the harms done by poverty. Such a perspective emerges from multiple sources, including the clinical work of Judith Herman, who iden-tified the origins of adult self-destructive behaviour in childhood sexual and physical abuse (van der Kolk *et al.* 1991, Herman 1992). But it also has origins in Indigenous scholarship, which elucidates the ongoing effects of colonisation and dispossession on individuals and communities (Fast and Collin-Vézina 2010, Purdie *et al.* 2014). Its influence has grown in the last few decades. 'Trauma-informed' barely existed as a descriptor of social welfare practice before 2000; but the Social Sciences Citation Index records 134 references for 2016 alone. Scholarly use of the term is dwarfed by practice and policy documents. In Australia, guidelines on trauma-informed care have been produced by national organisations rep-resenting mental health, child protection and family support, and govern-ment agencies direct service providers to build trauma-informed care into their practice. Yet the notion of 'trauma-informed' extends beyond service delivery. The Royal Commission into Institutional Responses to Child Sexual Abuse in Australia produced a discussion paper on trauma-informed care for victim-survivors of child sexual abuse (Quadara and Hunter 2016); the lead Commissioner, Justice McClellan (2015), has also called for trauma-informed justice. Moreover, the scope of 'trauma' has broadened from Herman's early work. Herman analysed complex trauma reactions in specific circumstances, that is, people who had been subject to sustained sexual abuse at critical developmental periods, at the hands of someone who had the victim under their control. In contrast, current homelessness services guidelines direct practitioners to embed trauma-informed care into usual practice, listing domestic violence, witnessing alcoholism and severe mental illness as risks (NSW Family and Com-munity Services 2014).

Trauma-based accounts both build on and depart from other ways of describing people who experience poverty. Historically, analyses of agency, whether progressive or conservative, have posited a more or less rational actor, acting under intention. Sociologists of the welfare subject, such as Fiona Williams, describe people as making rational choices within constraints: 'complexly and multiply positioned, engaged with, and acting upon, the diverse policy landscapes they inhabit' (Williams and Popay 1999, p. 159). Underclass theorists also argue for rational behaviour but claim that this rationality has perverse origins and consequences: Murray (1990) and Perkins (cited in Meloni 2016) argue that the welfare state rewards anti-social and pathological behaviour, and so has created people who behave pathologically because in the circumstances this is the rational way to behave. Trauma-informed accounts go further in describing behaviours as a self-preserving response to harm. The logic of trauma-informed care is that poverty is damaging and (some of) the poor are ineluctably *different* from the norm because they are damaged. The difference between underclass/undeserving poor accounts and trauma accounts is not the analytic frame, that is, the individual or social, but the locus of concern. Trauma-informed care makes calls on governments to address the circumstances in which trauma happens; conservative accounts also call on governments, but they call on them to dismantle the welfare state. Underclass accounts are concerned with the harm that the poor are doing to society, trauma accounts with the harms that have been done to the poor. Both, however, operate from the premise that agency is important, and that the agency of the poor is driven by deficiency.

The political implications of this dovetailing have attracted relatively little attention in scholarship of social policy or the welfare state. Other arenas of scholarship, however, which approach these questions of agency from a slightly different angle, can illuminate these considerations of poverty and practical justice.

Theorising justice and poverty, reprised: desire

So far, I have argued that studies of poverty which pay attention to experience converge in one important respect. Although they differ in their analysis of cause, effect and remedy, they share a concern with individual agency, and an understanding that the agency of the poor not in terms of bounded rationality or class habitus, but as dysfunction or damage. Although not explicitly framed in terms of identity politics, their shared concern with agency and difference draw from and extend this field, and two critical accounts of identity politics are especially useful here.

From the vantage of critical legal studies, Wendy Brown (1995) has studied the basis on which claims of harm can be made. Making use of the

Foucauldian analytic that power produces social identities which are then available for both politicisation and regulation, she argues that the concept of 'rights' is the mechanism by which the double movement of producing and constraining political advocacy is deployed. An example can be found in the welfare state, which produces welfare rights and the categories of people to whom those rights belong – such as mothers, people with disability, and people living in poverty. These categories, she argues, are therefore produced by both the idea of liberal justice and the reality in which that justice always fails (Brown 1995, p. 58). Brown takes issue with identity politics not because of its claims to difference, but because the conditions of its formation require a model of deficit. Its claims for justice are always based on the standard of a white masculine middle-class ideal, and on damage that has been done. In doing so, it binds claims for justice to social categories and enacts 'a politics of recrimination that seeks to avenge the hurt even while it reaffirms it, discursively codifies it' (Brown 1995, p. 74).

As an alternative, she proposes that the fixed category of identity be replaced by that of desire:

> What if we sought to supplant the identity of 'I am' – with its defensive closure on identity, its insistence on the fixity of position, its equation of social with moral positioning – with the language of 'I want this for us'? (This is an 'I want' that … [figures] a political or collective good as its desire.) What if we were to rehabilitate the memory of desire – either 'to have' or 'to be' – prior to its wounding?
>
> (Brown 1995, p. 75)

The Indigenous studies theorist Eve Tuck also lays claim to desire as a mechanism for claims to justice. She argues that 'damage-centred research', while politically and historically salient, constrains political agency and outcomes (Tuck 2009). Damage-centred research, her argument suggests, differs from 'deficit' models of poverty and disadvantage, such as those constructed by Murray and others, in two significant ways. First, it 'looks to historical exploitation, domination, and colonisation to explain contemporary brokenness, such as poverty, poor health, and low literacy' (Tuck 2009, p. 413). Second, it is distinct from conservative agency-based accounts of poverty in its intent. Rather than arguing that the state should protect itself from the poor, it makes claims on their behalf. Damage-based research operates 'from a theory of change that establishes harm or injury in order to achieve reparation' (Tuck 2009, p. 413).

The establishment of harm is a powerful means by which to seek redress, and an important part of claims to justice in civil and criminal arenas. However, Tuck argues, it exacts costs on those people who have already been harmed, including Indigenous people:

It is a powerful idea to think of us all as litigators, putting the world on trial, but *does it actually work?* Do the material and political wins come through? And, most importantly, are the wins worth the long-term costs of *thinking of ourselves as damaged?*

(Tuck 2009, p. 415)

Like Brown, Tuck looks to desire rather than harm as a means for animating claims to justice. Desire, she argues, has more dimensions than damage because it is concerned with 'complexity, contradiction and the self-determination of lived lives' (Tuck 2009, p. 416), and so is a better means for both understanding how people live and how things could be different.

Michelle Murphy draws these threads of damage and desire into her project, 'Alterlife' (2016). Her specific focus is on environmental politics and Indigenous justice, but the concept of alterlife has broad parameters and uses. Alterlife is that which has been altered, for example by 'human-invented chemicals […] settler colonialism, racism, and capitalism' (Murphy 2016, para. 2). The environmental and political damage done to Indigenous communities (Murphy's empirical focus is the Great Lakes region in the northern USA, but the circumstances she describes apply to Indigenous communities everywhere) is enormous, and this harm inheres in bodies at both the cellular and the social level. It is inevitable, and necessary, that this damage is known and named, since 'contemporary environmental politics is replete with apocalyptic anxieties, and descriptions of doomed and damaged communities' (Murphy 2016, para. 2). Nevertheless, she argues, affected communities also produce counter-narratives to these doomsday accounts, and the concept of alterlife recognises the fact that the lives that have already been changed are also open to future alteration. Rather than framing the future in terms of reparation for harm done, she calls for a reframing of biological difference and its 'entanglement within larger histories and geographies' (Murphy 2016, para. 2). How, she asks, 'might an investigation of alterlife as a shared, entangling, and yet unevenly distributed condition reframe and mobilize politics?' (Murphy 2016, para. 2). Alterlife, like desire, therefore is oriented towards counter-histories and alternative futures than those which rely on deviance from a standard, and reparation for harm.

Conclusion

I began this chapter with a discussion of poverty and the welfare state, and ended up with theorising of desire and identity. This may seem a recapitulation of old discussions in which questions of economic distribution are considered alongside questions of agency, only for one to be treated as more important than the other. Indeed, my focus on the undeserving poor, a group which is easily recognised but loosely defined, could be argued to be not really 'about' poverty at all: this is Murray's argument, that the underclass is characterised not by poverty but by social disorganisation. Yet generations of research show that the effects of poverty are not simply economic and that poverty is perpetuated by the mechanisms of large-scale social institutions (schools, social security systems) and everyday practices. Just as importantly, decades of research on the delivery of human services show that interventions intended to ameliorate disadvantage founder or thrive on their connection with the everyday agency of those they target. Addressing poverty in rich countries is a question of economic and social intervention, and while the two spheres are imbricated, as Butler argues, they are not, as Fraser argues, identical.

Brown, Tuck and Murphy share a concern with the basis on which claims for justice can be articulated and advanced, and are useful for thinking about practical justice for the undeserving poor in three ways. First, each recognises the significant harm that has been done to those who can make those claims, but also that people who have always already been changed are also open to further alteration. These harms are not trivial, but nor do they preclude agency or participation. Second, their accounts are based on difference but not deficiency. This allows for a stance distinct from that of the rational actor constructed in conventional accounts of public discourse, a construction which excludes those who apparently act against their best interests. Third, these accounts proceed from the entanglement of agency and structure. States, communities, politics, individual agency and collective desire are co-constitutive. Together, they present a way for thinking about participation and change that builds on social policy and social movements.

Lest this seem too cosy and conciliatory, it is worth noting that this form of securing practical justice will likely be expensive, requiring expenditure on both structure and agency. In terms of economics, the costs of policies to realistically address the harms that have been to generations of poor communities are likely to be substantial. Social policy tends sometimes to optimism about the transformative potential of one type of intervention or another: early childhood, or co-design, or behavioural economics. This is the type of optimism that says that it is possible for a well-designed and inexpensive intervention to return social and economic benefits for years to come. It is, in other words, a form of magical thinking (Brooks-Gunn 2003). Consider child protection, one of the most pressing 'wicked problems' of social policy. Protecting children in risky environments while preserving their families and supporting their parents is possible, but difficult, and more expensive than is often recognised in policy design. The programmes that are in place cannot help everyone who needs them, and moreover are designed in such a way that their failure to help can be blamed on families themselves for failing to engage. Facilitating the real participation of families in reconceptualising what safety and thriving can look like, and in defining and pursuing 'this is what we want', would be significantly more expensive than the conventional models of 'consultation' currently employed. Similar observations can be made about the failure of school systems to support the most marginalised, and the real costs needed to deliver the same quality of education to disadvantaged children as is currently delivered to the most privileged.

In terms of the social (or agency), it is not for nothing, I think, that Brown and Tuck turn to 'desire' rather than a less libidinally charged term. Desire has energies that overspill the boundaries of a Habermasian public sphere. From Freud to Delueze, desire invokes social connections and constructions, *and their opposite*, in the form of negativity and conflict (see Wilson 2015). Bringing desire into play animates the unconscious and affective dimensions of inequality and the work needed to address it: Fraser's description of 'subaltern counterpublics' recalls Spivak's (1988) deconstructive post-colonial readings of consciousness and subjectivity. The reviling of the undeserving poor serves the same cultural function as the Othering of racialised and sexualised difference – and many Indigenous people and communities bear the injuries of doubled marginalisation and stigmatisation. Efforts towards justice for those who are scapegoats for economic inequality, those who are called bludgers and junkies, must engage with the role that scapegoats play in keeping the rest of society comfortable. Claims to practical justice, in other words, and the participation of those who have been sidelined and stigmatised, is necessarily a claim to politics rather than technical questions of distribution.

References

Bourdieu, P., 1999. *The Weight of the World: Social Suffering in Contemporary Society.* Trans. P. P. Ferguson. Cambridge: Polity Press.
Bourgois, P., 1995. *In Search of Respect: Selling Crack in El Barrio.* Cambridge and New York: Cambridge University Press.
Brooks-Gunn, J., 2003. Do You Believe in Magic? What We Can Expect from Early Childhood Intervention Programs. *Social Policy Report*, 27 (1), 3–14.
Brown, W., 1995. *States of Injury: Power and Freedom in Late Modernity.* Princeton, NJ: Princeton University Press.
Butler, J., 1998. Merely Cultural. *New Left Review*, 227, 33–44.
Deacon, A., 2004. Different Interpretations of Agency within Welfare Debates. *Social Policy and Society*, 3 (4), 447–455. doi: 10.1017/S147474640400209X.
Desmond, M., 2016. *Evicted: Poverty and Profit in the American City.* New York: Penguin Random House.
Edin, K. J. and Shaefer, H. L., 2015. *$2.00 a Day: Living on Almost Nothing in America.* Boston: Houghton Mifflin Harcourt.
Fast, E. and Collin-Vézina, D., 2010. Historical Trauma, Race-based Trauma and Resilience of Indigenous Peoples: A Literature Review. *First Peoples Child & Family Review*, 5 (1), 126–136.

Fine, M., 1995. The Politics of Who's 'at Risk'. In: B. B. Swadner and S. Lubeck, eds, *Children and Families 'at Promise': Deconstructing the Discourse of Risk.* Albany: State University of New York Press, 76–94.

Fraser, N., 1995. From Redistribution to Recognition? Dilemmas of Justice in a 'Post-socialist' Age. *New Left Review*, 212, 68–93.

Fraser, N., 1997. Rethinking the Public Sphere: A Contribution to the Critique of Actually Existing Democracy. In: N. Fraser, ed., *Justice Interruptus: Critical Reflections on the 'Postsocialist' Condition.* New York and London: Routledge, 69–98.

Fraser, N. and Honneth, A., 2003. *Redistribution or Recognition? A Political-Philosophical Exchange.* London: Verso.

Fraser, N., Dahl, H. M., Stoltz, P. and Willig, R., 2004. Recognition, Redistribution and Representation in Capitalist Global Society: An Interview with Nancy Fraser. *Acta Sociologica*, 47 (4), 374–382.

Gornick, J. and Jäntti, M., 2014. *Income Inequality: Economic Disparities and the Middle Class in Affluent Countries.* Stanford: Stanford University Press.

Habermas, J., 1989 [1962]. *The Structural Transformation of the Public Sphere: An Inquiry into a Category of Bourgeois Society.* Trans. T. Burger. Cambridge: Polity.

Haylett, C., 2003. Culture, Class and Urban Policy: Reconsidering Equality. *Antipode*, 35 (1), 55–73.

Herman, J. L., 1992. Complex PTSD: A Syndrome in Survivors of Prolonged and Repeated Trauma. *Journal of Traumatic Stress*, 5 (3), 377–391. doi: 10.1007/bf00977235.

Jones, G. S., 2013. *Outcast London: A Study in the Relationship between Classes in Victorian Society.* London: Verso Books.

Katz, M. B., 2013. *The Undeserving Poor: America's Enduring Confrontation with Poverty.* 2nd edition. New York: Oxford.

Lansley, S. and Mack, J., 2015. *Breadline Britain: The Rise of Mass Poverty.* London: Oneworld Publications.

Levitas, R., 1998. *The Inclusive Society? Social Exclusion and New Labour.* Basingstoke: Palgrave.

McClellan, P., 2015. *Broken Structures, Broken Selves: Complex Trauma in the 21st Century.* Paper presented at the International Society for the Study of Trauma and Dissociation. Sydney: Royal Commission into Institutional Responses to Child Sexual Abuse.

Mead, L., 2013. The New Politics of the New Poverty. In: C. Pierson, F. G. Castles and I. K. Naumann, eds, *The Welfare State Reader.* Cambridge: Polity, 107–117.

Meloni, M., 2016. Welfare Poison: Why Everything You Believed about the Politics of Nature-Nurture May No Longer Be True. *Discover Society.* Available from: http://discoversociety.org/2016/07/05/welfare-poison-why-everything-you-believed-about-the-politics-of-nature-nurture-may-no-longer-be-true/.

Murphy, M., 2016. Alterlife in the Ongoing Aftermaths of Chemical Exposure. Available from: https://technopolitics.wordpress.com/technoscience-meets-biopolitics/.

Murray, C., 1990. *The Emerging British Underclass.* London: IEA.

Murray, C., 2013. *Coming Apart: The State of White America, 1960–2010.* New York: Crown Forum.

Murray, C. J. L., Kulkarni, S. C., Michaud, C., Tomijima, N., Bulzacchelli, M. T., Iandiorio, T. J., Ezzati, M. and Novotny, T., 2006. Eight Americas: Investigating Mortality Disparities across Races, Counties, and Race-Counties in the United States. *PLOS Medicine*, 3 (9), e260. doi: 10.1371/journal.pmed.0030260.

NSW Family and Community Services, 2014. *Specialist Homelessness Services: Practice Guidelines*. Sydney: NSW Family and Community Services.

Peel, M., 2003. *The Lowest Rung: Voices of Australian Poverty*. Cambridge, New York, Port Melbourne, Madrid, Cape Town: Cambridge University Press.

Piketty, T., 2014. *Capital in the 21st Century*. Trans. A. Goldhammer. Cambridge, MA: Belknap.

Purdie, N., Dudgeon, P. and Walker, R., 2014. *Working Together: Aboriginal and Torres Strait Islander Mental Health and Wellbeing Principles and Practice*. 2nd edition. Available from: www.telethonkids.org.au/our-research/early-environment/developmental-origins-of-child-health/aboriginal-maternal-health-and-child-development/working-together-second-edition/.

Quadara, A. and Hunter, C., 2016. *Principles of Trauma-informed Approaches to Child Sexual Abuse: A Discussion Paper*. Sydney: Royal Commission into Institutional Responses to Child Sexual Abuse. Available from: www.childabuseroyalcommission. gov.au/media-releases/discussion-paper-trauma-informed-approaches-child-sexual-abuse-released.

Rawls, J., 1958. Justice as Fairness. *Philosophical Review*, 67 (2), 164–194.

Saunders, P., 2015. Poverty and Social Disadvantage: Measurement, Evidence and Action. In: Committee for Economic Development of Australia, ed., *Addressing Entrenched Disadvantage in Australia*. Melbourne: CEDA, 21–32.

Shildrick, T., MacDonald, R. and Furlong, A., 2016. Not Single Spies but in Battalions: A Critical, Sociological Engagement with the Idea of So-called 'Troubled Families'. *Sociological Review*, 64 (4), 821–836.

Skeggs, B., 2011. Imagining Personhood Differently: Person Value and Autonomist Working-class Value Practices. *Sociological Review*, 59 (3), 496–513.

Spivak, G., 1988. Can the Subaltern Speak? In: C. Nelson and L. Grossberg, eds, *Marxism and the Interpretation of Culture*. Champaign, IL: University of Illinois Press, 271–316.

Swadener, B. B. and Lubeck, S., 1995. *Children and Families 'at Promise': Deconstructing the Discourse of Risk*. New York: State University of New York Press.

Tuck, E., 2009. Suspending Damage: A Letter to Communities. *Harvard Educational Review*, 79 (3), 409–427.

valentine, k., 2015. Complex Needs and Wicked Problems: How Social Disadvantage Became Multiple. *Social Policy and Society*, 15 (2), 237–249.

van der Kolk, B. A., Perry, J. C. and Herman, J. L., 1991. Childhood Origins of Self-destructive Behavior. *American Journal of Psychiatry*, 148 (12), 1665–1671.

Welshman, J., 2004. The Unknown Titmuss. *Journal of Social Policy*, 33 (2), 225–247.

Williams, F. and Popay, J., 1999. Balancing Polarities: Developing a New Framework for Welfare Research. In: F. Williams, J. Popay and A. Oakley, eds, *Welfare Research: A Critical Review*. London: UCL Press, 156–183.

Wilson, E. A., 2015. *Gut Feminism*. Durham, NC: Duke University Press.

Chapter 7

Engaging global institutions to achieve practical justice

The case of sexual rights

Sofia Gruskin and Alexandra Nicholson

Introduction

Practical justice is an all-encompassing term and can mean many things. As employed here, we conceptualise the term to imply an emphasis on fairness and equality, and at a practical level to include also a focus on accountability and actions to ensure that all populations, even those who are traditionally marginalised and discriminated against, are equally supported, engaged and counted. For this to occur at scale requires not only a vibrant civil society, but ultimately the financial and political commitment of every country in the world. Despite its obvious limitations, there is no place more important for understanding the collective concerns of countries as well as ensuring their financial and political commitment than the work of the United Nations (UN). Three overlapping streams of work at play within and across its institutions can be seen to shape much of the current global landscape. These can loosely be defined as the technical, the legal and the political. As used here, the technical stream covers the norms and standards developed by international technical agencies such as the World Health Organization (WHO) and the Joint United Nations Programme on HIV and AIDS (UNAIDS). Within the legal stream fall the formal parts of the human rights system including the Office of the High Commissioner for Human Rights (OHCHR), the United Nations treaty monitoring bodies, formal mechanisms such as special rapporteurs, as well as international court decisions. The political stream includes international government processes, with particular emphasis on the agreements made by states as these play out at the global level, as mostly recently seen in UN General Assembly agreements around the Sustainable Development Goals (SDGs). To support social movements in their efforts to facilitate change through the use of global-level spaces, this chapter sets out to offer some understanding of the language and approaches favoured by these different streams.

The chapter will use the issue of sexual rights specifically to demonstrate how these streams move forward independently, and yet overlap and draw strength from one another. These overlapping streams, each with their own histories, can be seen to shape much of the current global land-scape around sexual rights. They have a significant influence on one another, but they are distinct in orientation, practices and priorities. By naming them in this way, we hope to show how these distinctions influence the how and the why of the advances and retrenchments that occur in recognising and realising sexual rights, and how this awareness may be of use in advancing other issues of concern to practical justice.

There has never in history been such an opening up, both societally and legally, to the range of things we can understand to fall under the rubric of sexual rights. This includes an unprecedented number of countries accepting same-sex marriage, and at a minimum acknowledging the existence of lesbian, bisexual, gay, transgender and queer populations within their borders. This also includes growing recognition of sexual assault as a serious crime not only in the media, but by many governments. Nonetheless, there is simultaneously a growing backlash occurring against many aspects of sexual rights from all corners of the world, including not only outright violence and articulations of homophobia in communities and by many governments, but also retrenchment on commitments to good-quality comprehensive sexuality education, and to other aspects of sexual rights once thought not to be so contentious.

As with all topics, to begin to untangle what is good or bad about today's landscape for sexual rights requires attention to definitions, and ultimately to how sexual rights denote very different things depending on the actor and the context. It also requires an understanding of how the nature of the concern with specific topics (ranging from abortion to sexual orientation to sex work) influences the extent to which different actors engage in expansive or restrictive approaches. While resistance to sexual rights in many cases stems from claims to radically different understandings (and fears) of what 'sexual rights' includes, and therefore for states and others what it might bind them to, what is apparent in current debates is the way in which even those with an ostensibly expansive view of sexual rights in one domain may not have that same expansive perspective when it comes to other issues. The landscape of sexual rights, their definitions, as well as the standards promulgated by health and development organisations, human rights bodies and in political spaces, therefore, requires attention not only to what is included on websites and in publications, but also what has happened in recent history, within political currents and across social movements.

Sexual rights in technical spaces

Broadly speaking, as noted above, the technical stream as used here covers concepts, norms, standards, materials and guidelines developed by international agencies such as the WHO, UNAIDS and the United Nations Fund for Population Activities (UNFPA). Using the WHO as an example, the WHO uses 'evidence', including not only scientific evidence but legal definitions generated by the international human rights system and global political agreements, to give shape and support to sexual rights, and it does so because sexual rights are seen as necessary to achieve sexual health. In the context of sexual rights, actors on the technical side therefore tend to bring both human rights and law into their work because each matters for health outcomes, not because they are seen as important in their own right.

This approach has ultimately resulted in organisational acceptance of sexual rights not as a rights-affirming exercise, but as a practical reality necessary for the delivery and use of services which are the mainstay of the WHO's work and reason for being. And yet its work in this area, including the widely used working definition of sexual rights made publicly available on the WHO website (WHO 2010), gives legitimacy, support and 'evidence' for use by actors in many other spaces who are seeking to advance sexual rights and justice.

Below we examine how the definition of sexual rights within this space has progressed, as this may provide important insights as to how change can be facilitated in technical spaces.

The first written WHO-related formulation conceptualising sexual rights and what they entailed can be found in a WHO European Region technical document published in 1987. The document flagged the importance of the legal and policy environment to underpin the rights of individuals related to sexuality. It stated:

> Some positive concept of individual needs, responsibilities and rights in the area of sexuality needs to be established in order that laws that repress human rights can be changed (such as those against homosexuality or abortion) and that policies may be implemented to reduce restrictions on sexual expression and enable services to be established to deal with sexual problems.
>
> (WHO 1987)

It is important to note that the 1987 document, similar to documents produced by the WHO today, frames the importance of sexual health and rights and the need to address repressive laws and policies, not because they are discriminatory or harmful generally, but because of the need to establish health services to 'deal with sexual problems'.

More than a decade later, in 2000, the Pan American Health Organization (PAHO, which also serves as the WHO Regional Office for the Americas) and the World Association for Sexology (WAS) convened a regional consultation to examine how best to promote sexual health. Elaborated from an advocacy and policy standpoint, and very much fuelled by the HIV pandemic, it described three terms related to sexual health: sex, sexuality and sexual rights (PAHO 2000, p. 10). Out of this regional consultation it was agreed that '... since protection of health is a basic human right, it follows that sexual health involves sexual rights' (PAHO 2000, p. 10).

Here, the importance of sexual rights is placed within the context of the protection of sexual health. It is important to note that this was the first clear articulation of how human rights are thought to be relevant to sexual health. In examining how to move forward issues of practical justice in partnership with such technical organisations, the orientation of this statement is illustrative: in many ways this approach still drives the strategies around progressing sexual rights taken by the WHO and other actors working in this stream.

Several years later, in 2002, the WHO convened an international consultation to examine barriers to the promotion of sexual health. Participants at the consultation built on the work of the PAHO-WAS report and agreed upon working definitions of: sex, sexuality, sexual health and sexual rights, which were subsequently posted on the WHO website. This working definition of sexual rights is anchored in definitions from the legal stream, including UN human rights treaties, and the political stream, in particular the consensus documents of the 1994 International Conference on Population and Development (ICPD) (also referred to as 'Cairo') (ICPD 1994) and the Beijing Platform for Action from the Fourth World Conference on Women in 1995 (also referred to as 'Beijing') (UN Women 2014), as detailed below:

> Sexual rights embrace human rights that are already recognised in national laws, international human rights documents and other consensus statements. They include the right of all persons, free of coercion, discrimination and violence, to:
>
> - the highest attainable standard of sexual health, including access to sexual and reproductive health care services;
> - seek, receive and impart information related to sexuality;
> - sexuality education;
> - respect for bodily integrity;
> - choose their partner;
> - decide to be sexually active or not;
> - consensual sexual relations;
> - consensual marriage;
> - decide whether or not, and when, to have children; and
> - pursue a satisfying, safe and pleasurable sexual life.
>
> The responsible exercise of human rights requires that all persons respect the rights of others.
>
> (WHO 2006)

The 2002 definition has since progressed to a more inclusive definition, reproduced below. The updated 2006 definition which currently remains on the WHO website, in keeping with what came before, adopts an instrumental approach to sexual rights. It states:

> Sexual health is a state of physical, emotional, mental and social well-being in relation to sexuality; it is not merely the absence of disease, dysfunction or infirmity. Sexual health requires a positive and respectful approach to sexuality and sexual relationships, as well as the possibility of having pleasurable and safe sexual experiences, free of coercion, discrimination and violence. For sexual health to be attained and maintained, the sexual rights of all persons must be respected, protected and fulfilled.
>
> The fulfilment of sexual health is tied to the extent to which human rights are respected, protected and fulfilled. Sexual rights embrace certain human rights that are already recognized in international and regional human rights documents and other consensus documents and in national laws.
>
> Rights critical to the realization of sexual health include:
>
> - the rights to equality and non-discrimination
> - the right to be free from torture or to cruel, inhumane or degrading treatment or punishment
> - the right to privacy
> - the rights to the highest attainable standard of health (including sexual health) and social security
> - the right to marry and to found a family and enter into marriage with the free and full consent of the intending spouses, and to equality in and at the dissolution of marriage
> - the right to decide the number and spacing of one's children
> - the rights to information, as well as education
> - the rights to freedom of opinion and expression, and
> - the right to an effective remedy for violations of fundamental rights.
>
> The responsible exercise of human rights requires that all persons respect the rights of others.
>
> The application of existing human rights to sexuality and sexual health constitute sexual rights. Sexual rights protect all people's rights to fulfill and express their sexuality and enjoy sexual health, with due regard for the rights of others and within a framework of protection against discrimination.
>
> (WHO 2006)

While to some degree forward-looking, this often-cited technical definition, like those before it, has an explicit connection to health, thus rendering sexual rights simply a means towards improving health, and not an end in and of itself. Also worth noting is the fact that even as it appears on the WHO website, it is specifically called a 'working definition' rather than simply a 'definition', thus limiting its legitimacy if ever challenged (WHO 2010).

The evolution of the definition of sexual rights within this space shows that in working to advance practical justice claims in partnership with such technical organisations, it may be that the most useful way to progress is not to focus on rights and justice claims per se, but instead on the promotion of, or impediment to, rights *as they impact health outcomes*. One can see how this orientation would be extremely important from a strategic perspective to framing issues within technical spaces, even as this instrumental approach to advancing rights concerns may be frustrating to many engaged in social movements.

Understanding this progression and the way this definition has evolved sheds light on the need to understand why changes historically occur, including how terms are defined, where this has been documented, if and how changes were agreed upon, what pieces were controversial, and so on. Each is a distinct but vital point key to moving issues of practical justice forward within technical spaces.

Finally, on a practical level, in addition to the importance of framing rights claims in the context of health outcomes and understanding the importance of the historical evolution of terms, in partnering with technical organisations it is important to recall always the need to provide empirical evidence. For example, when interested in promoting the use of accountability mechanisms for health in this forum, it will be important to use on-the-ground evidence of where accountability mechanisms have mattered for health, and international legal and political consensus documents that demonstrate that this concept is not new but already well established.

Sexual rights in legal spaces

As defined here, the legal stream includes the formal parts of the human rights system, in particular the Office of the High Commissioner for Human Rights (OHCHR), the United Nations treaty monitoring bodies, and other formal mechanisms such as special rapporteurs. It also includes international and regional court decisions, as well as the United Nations Human Rights Council and other quasi-legal/political processes.

In the international legal arena, a trend can be seen whereby the focus of sexual rights tends to be on the respect, protection, fulfilment – and violation – of specifically articulated human rights as connected to sexuality. The focus again tends not to be on sexual rights per se. In this context, the emphasis is generally on non-discrimination and the right to be free from violence on the basis of sexual orientation (and to some degree gender identity), as well as the importance of law as it connects to sexuality, with minimal attention given to specific topical areas in sexual health or sexual rights in and of themselves. Furthermore, similar to the technical stream, in the legal sphere, health issues have been a strategic entry point to progress issues around sexual rights, particularly in the wake of the HIV pandemic. Using health as an entry point, there have been major advances for sexual rights, for example in relation to sexual orientation and to abortion, often justified even in this forum as necessary for public health.

It is important to note that when the words sexual (although almost always systematically alongside the word reproductive) rights are used in the legal space, the focus tends to primarily be on women, and women who are assumed to be in heterosexual sexual relationships. For example, unsafe abortion and its discriminatory and negative health impacts on women has been increasingly addressed by special rapporteurs, human rights treaty bodies and other actors in the legal sphere as a matter of sexual and reproductive health and rights (CEDAW 2011, Grover 2011). While this may be frustrating for those engaged with practical justice initiatives, knowing the limitations within this space is key to understanding and working with partner organisations in legal spaces.

Overall, UN treaty monitoring bodies have been increasingly giving attention to the application of international human rights law to various dimensions of sexuality, such as autonomy, non-discrimination and equality, accountability, participation and empowerment and international cooperation in particular, even as none use the term 'sexual rights'. For example, in a recent General Comment put out by the UN Committee on Economic, Social and Cultural Rights, a 'right to sexual and reproductive health' is named (ESCR 2016). There have also been tentative advances in several special rapporteur reports (e.g. Grover 2011), even though only one has attempted a specific articulation of sexual rights (Hunt 2004). How one sees the relationship between sexual rights and human rights law is critically important in this stream; different actors distinguish in different ways whether sexual rights are considered implicit or explicit in existing human rights law. When sexual rights are considered to be explicit, this is critically important to identify given that law is enforceable regardless of how the term sexual rights is defined. This enforceability can be used as leverage for social movements in this space. Conversely, in instances where specific rights termed sexual rights or certain concepts around sexuality are not yet established internationally, and are therefore not yet legally enforceable, this lack of legal backing should be recognised and worked around accordingly.

In this vein, certain rights are advanced as sexual rights because they have resonance within particular country contexts for political, historical, societal and/or legal reasons. Legal gender identity recognition, for example, has been successfully and comprehensively addressed by Argentinean legislators in the context of the right to identity, as the right to identity is of major historical relevance within the country. In Germany, given its historical and political context, the right to be free from forceful medical interventions has great relevance, hence the right to self-determination and to bodily integrity has been evoked comprehensively in cases of forced sterilisations of transgender people. Recognising the historical context of each country is vital to progressing issues of practical justice via social movements. While fighting against decades of political, societal and legal norms is oftentimes necessary to advance issues of practical justice, familiarity with the history of the country within which the movement is working can help not only in domestic work but to explain positions being taken at the international level, and help in framing issues in ways they will be seen and heard within the legal stream.

Although in recent years the world has seen an unprecedented opening towards sexual rights in other domains, in the legal space the definition and progression of sexual rights claims appears narrow and constrained. Yet, there have been many advances with respect to protections and legal claims in the legal arena even if these have been around specific topics and themes. These distinctions matter for rights work in many ways. Worthy of particular note is the fact that social movements focused on addressing legal and policy restrictions around sexual behaviour (including same-sex practices) are not identical to the legal and policy efforts needed to defend various gendered behaviours and identities. Both may find resonance in the legal arena, but may be predicated on different groundings in different rights claims or concerns. While this is not necessarily a bad thing, the advocacy approaches of social movements pursuing topics of practical justice in the legal sphere are best served by ensuring explicit and concrete attention to a named population and to the naming of specific rights as enshrined in international human rights legal documents. Such attention is key to advancing issues of practical justice for social movements attempting to make change using the legal space.

Sexual rights in political spaces

As previously mentioned, the political stream generally includes international and regional government processes, with particular emphasis on global conferences and/or the international declarations made by states in these global-level forums. Despite its importance, it is often the least progressive space to work within. In this vein, moving concepts forward within the political stream will oftentimes be via a lowest common denominator approach, with progress made by offering up a point of agreement or consensus even if not far-reaching, so long as it is not retrogressive. Facilitating change in political spaces frequently relies on outside efforts by social movements that states in the political space react and respond to, including simply ensuring the documents coming out of any relevant events reflect technical and legal definitions which are seen as beyond question.

While advances at the political level are oftentimes painfully slow, when moving forward issues of practical justice it is important to realise how much these standards, once agreed upon, may be the most important of all. Once in place, political standards can be used to frame arguments that are more likely to be accepted by states and institutions of power within countries, and in ways that can facilitate access to resources which can then support technical and legal advances as well as directly support people's lived realities. The broad history of the progression of the concept of sexual rights in political spaces below helps illuminate several important strategies to keep in mind when pushing forward issues of practical justice in this space.

Sexual rights at the global political level, like the two streams noted above, started from sexual health as derivative of reproductive health, and is grounded in the International Conference on Population and Development (often called the Cairo consensus). This was, amongst other things, the first intergovernmental agreement that attempted to define sexual health. Importantly, this political articulation drew from a 1975 WHO technical report on human sexuality (WHO 1975, pp. 6–7). Ultimately, with respect to sexual rights, arguably no language has been as important as paragraph 96 of the 1995 Beijing Platform for Action. Despite numerous on-the-record reservations from a host of countries, paragraph 96, which appears in the health chapter of the Beijing document, states:

> The human rights of women include their right to decide freely and responsibly on all matters related to their sexuality, free of coercion, discrimination and violence.
>
> (UN 1995, p. 36)

This definition not only builds on the Cairo consensus, but grounds its articulation within the internationally agreed legal human rights framework. Furthermore, while the focus on women can now be seen as problematic for many reasons, it is important historically not to forget that this focus on the health and rights of women was at the time essential in moving global consensus beyond the need to control women's fertility as part of a demographic agenda with little attention to the impacts of decisions taken in these forums on the rights and health of women themselves. At the present moment there are other concerns with this definition we can point to: not only the fact that it is limited to women, but also its focus only on health in application and scope. Similar to the technical definitions discussed above, sexual rights are relevant only because of their implications for health. Nonetheless, this statement represents the first (and to this day perhaps the strongest) inter-governmentally agreed-to articulation of what have become known as sexual rights in this space.

Since Cairo and Beijing, the past two decades have shown an unprecedented expansion in both understanding and political articulations related to sexual rights. However, huge complexities have emerged, so that the current landscape of sexual rights is fraught with conundrums and sometimes insoluble questions. Overall, many countries currently express support for at least some aspects of statements put forth in the name of sexual rights, including rights in relation to sexual orientation and/or gender identity, but express their refusal to agree to the usage of the term 'sexual rights'. In this vein, countries oftentimes cite the legal and political ambiguity surrounding the term. Other countries declare that they do not support the term sexual rights because they do not agree with the content of sexual rights, even when undefined. At times countries justify this position based upon how the term sexual rights has been used in other political contexts.

Both the Cairo and Beijing conferences to this day remain touchstones undergirding sexual rights in all spheres. Interestingly, these political definitions, perhaps because they are ostensibly endorsed by a majority of the governments of the world, continue to be given space as the ultimate voice on the content, extent and existence of sexual rights, despite their obvious limitations. Acknowledging the limits of this political definition of sexual rights, particularly its explicit and exclusive focus on women, is important. Such weaknesses in political spaces are important to identify by those seeking to move forward issues of practical justice in all spheres, as they may signal points of contention and areas where progress is needed but may be difficult.

Certain rights are advanced as sexual rights in this space because they have resonance within particular country contexts because of political, historical, societal and/or legal tradition. Just like in the legal sphere, tracking the support or lack of support of human rights standards in various political spaces is another important means to realising practical justice; in instances where they are supported, human rights can be used to frame issues of practical justice in language that political actors understand. Those engaging in moving forward issues of practical justice in this space may wish to consider not only these complexities and differences in the perspectives offered by different countries, but also recognise that each of these articulations is important to progress in different contexts.

Furthermore, the distinction between sexual rights, as opposed to reproductive rights, sexual and reproductive rights, and sexual and reproductive health and rights continues to be another related area of express ambiguity in the political space. In cases where 'sexual and reproductive rights' are lumped together in one term, the boundaries between these two areas are often defined differently by various political actors. Take, for example, the Sustainable Development Goals (SDGs). Ultimately, the SDGs recognise sexual and reproductive health and rights in a rather awkward formulation. While there exist strong political commitments, there is an inconsistent use of relevant terminology (that is, the mismatch between the terms 'sexual' and 'reproductive' and simply reproductive in this goal) (UN 2017). This inconsistency in terminology has major implications for the targets and indicators set to measure country progress, with implications for the data to be collected by countries to show fulfilment of this goal. Therefore, what funding is available and for what programmes, even at the most local level, is impacted upon by the ambiguity of this language. Sometimes this type of ambiguity is the result of careful thought, but other times it is simply the result of political pressure. As can be seen through this example, identifying varying definitions and ambiguities within political documents, as well as recognising the intent, or lack thereof, behind them is vital to framing issues of practical justice in this space.

Integrated nature of the three streams

As can be seen from the above, the three streams have a significant influence on one another, although they are sufficiently distinct in orientation and priority. By naming the three streams in this way our intent is to distinguish between their unique influences, and identify the how and the why of the advances and retrenchments that are occurring in recognising and realising sexual rights within each space.

While each stream is distinct, they are also very much interconnected and, as shown in the above example, at the global level actors in each sphere often rely on the definitions in another stream to give legitimacy to the definition they put forth. For example, NGOs involved in lobbying global political processes related to sexual rights will often rely on the WHO working definition as the basis for their advocacy. As noted above, while the political represents the lowest common denominator across all spheres, legal definitions use the political and the technical definitions to undergird the legitimacy of any positions they stake out – particularly concerning the links between sexuality and human rights more generally. Overall, states and other actors tend to give weight to WHO documents and definitions in the political space precisely because they are assumed to be technical and evidence-based. Ultimately, the political environment plays a critical role in which issues are taken up and which are left aside in all spheres, including the technical and the legal.

For those working on the technical side, a strategy most apparent in the work of the WHO, 'evidence' includes legal and political definitions, and is used to give shape and support to the importance of sexual rights particularly as necessary for sexual health. Furthermore, the technical side uses human rights and law, and definitions articulated in the legal stream, in their work on sexual health because human rights and law matter for health outcomes – to reiterate, the focus is oftentimes not because of a concern with rights per se but because the promotion of, or impediment to, sexual rights has an impact on health outcomes. The emphasis on health exists to some degree in all three streams and reveals that, at least at this point in time, sexual and/or reproductive health for almost all actors in the global space is the justification for dealing with sexual rights, and not rights pertaining to sexuality for all people for their own sake. With the help of social movements focused on practical justice, recognition of this limitation can hopefully be addressed moving forward. For those engaged with actors in a particular stream working to progress issues of practical justice, it is crucial to recognise not only the distinct qualities of the space in which each is working, but also the ways in which previous progress or established definitions made in other streams can be used and applied to carry forward the work at hand.

Conclusion

Overall, the past two decades have shown an unprecedented expansion in understanding and standard-setting related to sexual rights at the global level in the technical, legal and political spheres. With these developments, however, huge complexities remain to be addressed. Understanding where progress has been made around this topic, and where backlash has occurred within each of the three streams, is relevant to the struggle to facilitate change around issues of practical justice.

Those engaging in actions to advance sexual rights must not only examine these conundrums and questions, but also recognise that each of these articulations is important in different contexts, taking into account current North/South, North/North and South/South politics at a governmental level, as well as what is happening with those opposed to sexual rights in all forums. In the current world of SDGs, the examples noted above may help us to consider how best to support a diverse sexual rights agenda, not only in terms of advocacy but in the programmatic work of international governmental organisations, multilateral and bilateral funding and state agencies.

It is important to note that there are a set of questions that can be derived from this example that will require attention and analysis, whatever the issue at stake. A potential first step can be to map, in order to make explicit, not only the (in)consistencies among the technical, legal and political areas, but also where there are gaps in standards relating to populations or topics that remain to be addressed. Such a mapping would make it easier to analyse where it would help to ensure consistency and where it might be strategic to let things be. Where standards do exist, there is a clear need to document the difference they have made to people's lives. Standards that have been put in place can effectively be used to frame arguments that are more likely to be accepted by states and institutions of power within countries, and in ways that can facilitate access to resources which can then further support direct impacts on people's lives.

This chapter has implications for all those concerned with practical justice, not only for people seeking to advance a sexual rights agenda. Although serious progress has been made in the last two decades, efforts are being made daily to weaken global solidarity and global principles and institutions, a concern for all social movements that make justice a priority. Equality, non-discrimination and universalism are key to all social movements working to achieve practical justice. It is of critical importance that these principles remain central to all work in this area. Fighting for practical justice within the broader negative geopolitical changes occurring requires forming and maintaining broad coalitions – ones aimed at preserving our web of international partnerships, from the people we work with, to how we work together, to how we understand the work we do within a framework of international relations and solidarity. Focusing on this kind of action is a matter of prudence to the work of practical justice; as individuals and as a collective group of human beings, we need to figure out how and when to act. This means that across the range of topics we work on we have to work together more actively between and across the technical, legal and political spaces identified here to support people to be able to claim their rights, and to protect people who advocate for these rights.

Who is vulnerable or disadvantaged clearly will vary between countries and within countries, but we need vigilance to ensure that a focus now and in the future results in better norms and standards within the technical, legal and political spaces in all areas of concern to those engaged in practical justice. We must all be concerned with ensuring greater support for the justice of all people, and how this translates into the lived experience of all people, everywhere in the world and without distinction.

Acknowledgement

With thanks to Peter Aggleton for his support throughout the preparation of this chapter, and to Jane Cottingham, Eszter Kismodi, Alice Miller and Sonia Correa for the initial discussion that led to to its preparation.

References

CEDAW, 2011. *Communication No. 22/2009, L. C. v. Peru.* New York: CEDAW. Available from: www2.ohchr.org/english/law/docs/CEDAW-C-50-D-22-2009_en.pdf.

ESCR, 2016. *The Right to Sexual and Reproductive Health (Article 12 of the International Covenant on Economic, Social and Cultural Rights).* New York: United Nations. Available from: http://tbinternet.ohchr.org/_layouts/treatybodyexternal/Download. aspx?symbolno=E%2fC.12%2fGC%2f22&Lang=en.

Grover, A., 2011. *Right of Everyone to the Enjoyment of the Highest Attainable Standard of Physical and Mental Health A/66/254.* New York: United Nations. Available from: https://documents-dds-ny.un.org/doc/UNDOC/GEN/N11/443/58/PDF/ N1144358.pdf?OpenElement.

Hunt, P., 2004. *Promotion and Protection of Human Rights: Human Rights Questions, Including Alternative Approaches for Improving the Effective Enjoyment of Human Rights and Fundamental Freedoms E/CN.4/2004/49.* New York: United Nations. Available from: https://documents-dds-ny.un.org/doc/UNDOC/GEN/G04/109/33/PDF/ G0410933.pdf?OpenElement.

ICPD, 1994. *Programme of Action of the International Conference on Population Development.* Cairo: United Nations Population Fund. Available from: www.unfpa.org/ sites/default/files/pub-pdf/programme_of_action_Web%20ENGLISH.pdf.

PAHO, 2000. *Promotion of Sexual Health: Recommendations for Action: Proceedings of a Regional Consultation Convened by the Pan American Health Organization and the World Health Organization in Collaboration with the World Association for Sexology.* Guatemala: PAHO. Available from: www1.paho.org/hq/dmdocuments/2008/ PromotionSexualHealth.pdf.

UN Women, 2014. *Beijing Declaration and Platform for Action: Beijing+5 Political Declaration and Outcome.* New York: UN Women. Available from: www2.unwomen. org/~/media/headquarters/attachments/sections/csw/pfa_e_final_web. pdf?v=1&d=20160316T150800.

United Nations, 1995. *Report of the Fourth World Conference on Women.* New York: United Nations. Available from: www.un.org/womenwatch/daw/beijing/pdf/ Beijing%20full%20report%20E.pdf.

United Nations, 2017. *Sustainable Development Goals.* Available from: www.un.org/ sustainabledevelopment/sustainable-development-goals/.

WHO, 1975. *Education and Treatment in Human Sexuality: The Training of Health Professionals. WHO Technical Report Series No. 572.* Geneva: World Health Organization. Available from: http://apps.who.int/iris/bitstream/10665/38247/1/ WHO_TRS_572_eng.pdf.

WHO, 1987. *Concepts of Sexual Health. Report of a Meeting in Copenhagen, May 1987.* Copenhagen: World Health Organization.

WHO, 2006. *Defining Sexual Health.* Geneva: World Health Organization. Available from: www.who.int/reproductivehealth/topics/sexual_health/sh_definitions/en/.

WHO, 2010. *Sexual and Reproductive Health: Defining Sexual Health.* Geneva: World Health Organization. Available from: www.who.int/reproductivehealth/topics/ sexual_health/sh_definitions/en/.

Part II

From principles to practice

Chapter 8

Practical justice in social work and social welfare

Contested values

Richard Hugman

Introduction: some historical fragments

Professional social work and the broader field of social welfare as this is now understood emerged in the nineteenth century in the countries of north-western Europe, Scandinavia and North America that had led the Industrial Revolution (Payne 2005). Historical analyses highlight developments in Denmark, the Netherlands, the UK and the USA as among the earliest leading to the provision of formalised professional social work and modern social welfare services (Healy 2008).

In the late 1800s the primary force for growth within the social welfare field came from responses to the poverty and disadvantage that were widespread in the rapidly expanding urban centres. One major strand of such responses was the effort by those who were involved in the provision of charitable assistance to harness the insights of science by creating 'scientific charity'. These were the Charity Organisation Societies (COS), which, among other things, originated the practice of casework. Through such an approach, charitable relief was targeted to those who could be identified scientifically as capable of making best use of it. To this was tied the acceptance of personal assistance to learn coping skills and ways of avoiding a return to poverty.

A second significant element of early social work is seen in the growth of hospital almoners. Like the COS, they were concerned with poverty and disadvantage at the level of individuals and families. However, their primary role was to help people who were too poor to access health care to do so through the allocation of charitable funds ('alms' as they were then called). The hospital almoners also mostly used 'casework' methods and principles. In some countries, such as Australia, hospital almoners constituted the largest of these early forms of professional social work.

The third strand came from the actions of political critics who sought to rectify what they saw as the structural origins of poverty and disadvantage. This approach coalesced around what became known as the settlement houses, which can be seen as the early form of community development. In these institutions, those with (what is now termed) social capital resided in the poorest districts to work together with members of those communities to seek improvements in living and working conditions. For example, Toynbee Hall in London was founded in 1884 by Samuel and Henrietta Barnett (Payne 2005). Their aim was to involve those training in universities and other members of the elite classes in social action against poverty. As well as providing advice and support to individuals, Toynbee Hall also established education programmes, community-based welfare for children and families, and campaigned for improvements in housing. Hull House, in Chicago, was founded in 1888 by Jane Addams after she visited Toynbee Hall and undertook similar work.

As Payne (2005) points out, not everyone who was affected by poverty was equally a subject of social work interest, but usually those who had a particular need for care or assistance beyond that which may be regarded as reasonably met by expectations that wherever possible people will care for themselves and their families. Thus the direct relief of poverty was often left to broader social welfare measures, combined with economic policies, while '[...] social work's clientele are not all those in poverty but specific sub-groups: children and families; elderly people; mentally ill people and people with physical and learning disabilities' (Payne 2005, p. 122).

Commenting on social work in the present day, England sees this thread continuing over time, although he expresses the point more generally in the observation that '[...] social work does not exist for people with problems, rather it helps people who cannot cope with their problems unaided' (England 1983, p. 13). In other words, social work within social welfare focuses on those people who are seen to be 'most in need'.

Thus, in the origins of social work and social welfare we can see the roots of debates and issues that continue over time. In summary, these can be regarded as aspects of the core debate about the extent to which poverty, disadvantage and other forms of social misery are produced by circumstances, individual incapacity and bad choices or the lack of opportunity, communal disadvantage and structural inequality. How these points are debated was variously influenced by social, political and religious ideologies. In short, this established the ongoing debate about whether poverty, disadvantage and social misery are matters of bad luck or of social injustice. While it can be said that, in broad terms, political differences between liberalism and socialism tend to mirror the distinction between individual and collective explanations of poverty and disadvantage, wider social, cultural and religious differences do not map so easily onto this binary distinction.

The twentieth-century development of social work and social welfare was greatly impacted upon by the two major international conflicts of the

Great War of 1914–18 and the World War of 1939–45. Both these major conflicts saw rapid shifts in the further professionalisation of social work and the emergence of the modern 'welfare state'. In the period 1918–39, for example, Australia saw the foundations being set for what became known as the 'wage earners' welfare state' (Castles 1994), while in the UK the Poor Law of 1601 finally gave way to an entitlement system of state pensions and benefits between 1930 and 1948 (Spicker 1988).

Two more factors need to be identified by way of introduction. The first of these is the internationalisation of social work and social welfare. In 1928, an International Committee of Social Workers (ICSW) met in Paris and established a committee on professional education (Healy 2008). The participants came from all perspectives in the field, sharing ideas and practice developments. Many were involved at governmental levels in their own countries in the formation of social welfare policies. This organisation was torn apart by political tensions in the late 1930s, and in the late 1940s and early 1950s struggled to reform, resulting in three organisations: the International Council on Social Welfare (ICSW), the International Association of Schools of Social Work (IASSW) and the International Federation of Social Workers (IFSW). Leading members of these organisations were also instrumental in establishing various significant bodies in the post-conflict world, including several of the United Nations entities (Seibel 2008).

Of particular note here is the transition of ICSW from identification with *social work* as a profession to *social welfare* as a field. In the earlier part of the twentieth century, social work was spread beyond the global North[1] through colonial systems of governance, with tertiary-level colleges being founded in India, Egypt and Buenos Aires. Ironically, these all pre-date the first university social work programme in Australia by almost a decade. Post-1945, in processes of decolonisation, the systems of social welfare and the formation of professional social work became part of the struggle for independence, so that in most African countries, for example, quite different models and systems have developed (for example, see Osei-Hwedie 1993). So, while in the global North social work came to represent the professionalisation of social welfare, in the global South this relationship is more tenuous so that concerns often rest with multi-disciplinary views of social welfare as a field.

Meanwhile, in the global North the ongoing process of professionalisation of social work continues to face issues of fuzzy boundaries, in that social work theories and practices often sit between those of other disciplines and professions and disciplines. While social work has provided numerous practice concepts to the wider field of social welfare, including casework, case management, social groupwork and so on, these have all in different ways been broadened to include those with other forms of professional education or members of other recognised professions.

However, social work has also brought to the wider social welfare field the early debates between individual bad luck and collective injustice in the formation of poverty, disadvantage and social misery, with implications for the choices to be made in structures, policies and practices as to how these phenomena should be addressed. This chapter considers this ongoing value debate through examining the role of social work in social welfare.

Rawls against Nozick – social welfare and the neo-liberal backlash

The developments in social work and social welfare that have been sketched out above must be understood in their social, political and cultural context. Wider debates that followed the end of the World War in 1945 tended to promote concern with peace-building, which was often embodied in policies aimed at constructing a better world for all those who had their lives impacted so severely. Indeed, these are often seen as the driving force of the different forms of welfare state that emerged across the global North (Spicker 1988, Esping-Andersen 1990).

Underlying these developments was a deeper value debate about the sort of post-war society that people sought. Social and political philosophy (like many disciplines including medicine and psychology) saw many arguments around the nature of society, the relationship between people, responsibility and so on, that extended older debates in the new circumstances. One of the most influential of his generation was the political philosopher John Rawls (1972), whose ideas impacted on more than a generation of global Northern social work and social welfare (for example, see Ferguson 2008, p. 32).

Rawls's basic premise is that wellbeing should not depend on luck (Hinman 2013). His argument is that much of what produces poverty, disadvantage and social misery has causes beyond any individual's immediate control. In corollary, the benefits enjoyed by those who avoid misery through wealth and advantage mostly accrue from things other than their own careful exercise of responsibility. Even talent, which may advantage some people over others, is not to our moral credit, according to Rawls.

Consequently Rawls (1972) proposed social rules designed to maximise fairness and minimise arbitrary benefit. These rules include the principle that inequality is only justified if it is in some way to the benefit of the least well-off. Thus inequality is most usually unjust because so often depends on being sustained by social rules that benefit people on the basis of factors over which they have no control, and therefore for which they can take no moral credit. In this way, justice concerns both sides of a balance of fairness, rather than simply being focused on one side that is perceived to be in deficit.

Over the decades, social work and social welfare have increasingly tended to operate on the basis of this understanding of social justice. In the most recent iteration of social work's ethical principles, social justice is regarded as one of the key organising values from which other ethics and value statements can be drawn (IFSW/IASSW 2004, AASW 2010). For example, Banks (2004, p. 80) at one point identified the idea of social justice solely with redistributive principles concerning access to material resources (although she has subsequently developed a much more nuanced and wider-ranging argument, see Banks 2012).

Against this position, Nozick (1974) argues that differences in wellbeing and social circumstances cannot be regarded as matters of justice, precisely because they are, indeed, simply matters of luck. Extending the much earlier notion (from Locke 1980 [1690]) that the right to property derives from mixing one's self with the natural world through labour, Nozick claims that injustice arises when a person is required to give up something in favour of another person unless that thing is freely given. This argument has two elements of relevance to the present discussion. First, for Nozick, inequality simply exists as a state of the natural world. On this basis it cannot be considered a moral issue. Second, to take a person's property for a purpose to which that person has not consented actually takes something of the person. Thus, taxation to fund social welfare is an injustice. In contrast, while charitable giving if freely done may be morally creditworthy, it is supererogatory and cannot be demanded.

Opponents of social welfare tend to invoke variations of Nozick's argument, to the effect that assistance that is provided through taxation comes at the expense of taking the property of others. In the USA, this has most recently taken the form of opposition to the so-called 'Obamacare' reforms in health. In Australia, it appears in public discourse as criticisms of 'bludgers' (most recently 'leaners') and in the UK of 'scroungers'. While this attack on publicly funded social welfare has the appearance of Locke's argument about personhood and property, it lacks his concern that accumulating more than one needs weakens the moral claim to property. In this, Locke appeared to be echoing the earlier Thomist argument that 'whatever a man [sic] has in superabundance is owed, of natural right, to the poor for their sustenance' (in Singer 2004, p. 185). In the twenty-first century, such other-directed concern combined with self-restraint, which it can be said marked the 'welfare consensus' of the post-1945 era, seems now to have left the stage.

Behind the practical language of bludgers is usually a question of 'desert' that was also part of some very early social work debates, especially among those involved in the COS movement and, to an extent, the hospital almoners. However, whereas the late-nineteenth-century judgement about deservingness was mixed with concern about the potential for the recipient of charity to make good use of it, so that such resources would be used to best effect, arguments about moral worthiness appear to have become separated even from this moderating notion, and in some debates could be said to have taken over the ethical underpinnings of social welfare completely. This process has seen the reappearance of the concern that only those whose need can be regarded as entirely a misfortune have a claim in the support of others. But added to older notions of the 'feckless poor', there are now concerns with other ways of questioning desert, such as whether welfare claimants carry other types of questionable social identity. Examples of such moral judgement to which this discussion returns below are those of people with disabilities and refugees and other migrants. In this sense, rather than a truly liberal position, the challenge to social welfare is more correctly understood as neo-liberalism and this in turn having a bond, at times under strain, with neo-conservatism that subtly connects anxieties over moral unworthiness with antagonism to social change (Hugman 1998, Ferguson 2008).

By the late 1990s it had become clear that the demise of a rough consensus that tended to favour Rawls rather than Nozick was placing social workers and other practitioners in social welfare under increasing pressure in their commitment to the core value of social justice as a foundation for their work (Hugman 1998). The dominance of neo-liberalism led to models of social welfare services that sought to recast them in a quasi-market mould, with practitioners as 'producers' and service users as 'consumers'. As part of this process there is a logic that in order to enable service users to exercise choice and at the same time take more responsibility for their own lives, the power of professionals should be restricted to that of technical competence, that is, determining how objectives prescribed by others are to be achieved. This shift removes one of the central claims of professionalism to setting broad value-based goals concerning the scope and purposes of their actions. While the rhetoric of such a change is that those setting goals will be service users, in reality the use of contracts and government regulation means that managers, policymakers and politicians have tended to assume the power of professionals rather than such power substantially being transferred to service users (Lymbery 2014).

Professions, power and social justice

Even within a neo-liberal environment, social workers and other actors in the social welfare field exercise considerable power in relation both to the framing of social need and the systems that respond to it. As practitioners they also exercise power directly in relation to service users, whether as individuals, families, groups or communities. Such power can take a number of forms (Hugman 1991), which include knowledge and skills that come from education, authority attached to social roles, and so on. Not only are social workers and other social welfare actors able to influence, at times even coerce, whether implicitly or explicitly, indi-viduals, families and social groups, they also play a part in setting the broader social agenda in which social welfare is enacted and even forming the language and ideas through which the reality of social need and welfare responses are shaped.

This understanding of social power presents a challenge to many social workers and others in social welfare, in so far as the overt purposes of these occupations is to meet needs and to provide 'care'. There are two major ways in which social workers and others have reacted to this: first, by reject-ing the implications of this analysis and seeking to reframe these professions so as to remove these dimensions (for example, see Ife 1997); second, by accepting this as inevitable, providing a certainty to the purposes of profes-sional action, and asserting the use of ethics to ensure that practice is dir-ected to meeting need. Ife's view is that to be true to its political and moral core, social work should sever its connections with service provision and ally itself with collective struggles to change policies and systems. In this, Ife is revisiting the radical aspects of the early settlement house movement, char-acterising the heart of social work as community development. The altern-ative position can be seen as 'orthodox' practice, rarely argued as such but played out in practice, policy and research that focus on how to meet the requirements of the current system effectively and ethically.

There is another possible position. Another range of commentators seek to find ways in which the necessary services (including that which might be seen as 'care') can be provided for those who need them, each arguing that this should be done in ways that pursue the social justice claims of social work. This position (or positions, as it includes a wide range of otherwise often subtly different arguments) draws on various the-ories and concepts, including neo-Marxism, critical psychoanalysis, post-modernism, environmentalism and (a return to) questions of spirituality (for example: Ferguson 2008, Alston 2009, Dominelli 2012, Gardner 2014, Besthorn *et al.* 2016). The commonality to these various arguments is a focus on how social workers and others in the social welfare field may address the needs of marginalised and disadvantaged people while at the same time seeking change in the structures and systems that exist to meet need but at the same time may create or exacerbate needs. In other words, can professional power be rethought so that it becomes the basis for the practical pursuit of social justice?

Practical cases: disability services and refugee settlement

To provide brief illustrations of the issues that these debates raise, I want to sketch out some implications by looking at services for people with dis-abilities and for refugees. These two examples are chosen specifically because, in his original discussion of justice, Rawls (1972) refers to people with disabilities and, it is alleged (Banerjee 2011), he excluded people such as refugees because of questions about citizenship (a point to which this discussion returns below). Both these groups are of great concern in social welfare in Australia.

In the area of disability services, over many years there has been a growing movement of service users seeking a strong voice. There are different approaches to this, of which here I will address two. The first of these can be understood in terms of a consumer model (Oliver *et al.* 2012). A consumer model considers the achievement of power by people with disabilities through creating mechanisms that allow control over the resources of care, with the service user taking the role of purchaser of care and other services. That is, through direct decision-making about the use of resources the disabled person or their family can exercise power by making direct decisions concerning their own lives. The logic is that professionals have tended to make decisions that ignore the interests of the disabled person or their family, often including directly expressed ideas and preferences. At the extreme, this position can regard professionals as in opposition to disabled people, with decisions being made in the interest of the professionals.

In comparison, the alternative approach regards professionals as potential allies and seeks to create partnerships to pursue appropriate care and support (Oliver *et al.* 2012). This way of responding to the power of professionals takes a different stance, one that seeks to change the relationship between service users and professionals such that power is shared (Postle and Beresford 2007). At the same time it requires professionals to consider that their knowledge and skills, use of access to institutions and so on are open to question. There is, in this, an ethical imperative, namely that accountability means being able to give an account, in this case to service users individually and collectively.

In some ways the area of care and support for refugees in a country of settlement raises comparable issues. Here too the power of professionals is crucial (Westoby 2009, Robinson 2014). What this means is that professionals assisting in the settlement process work in such a way as to open up their practices in sharing knowledge and skills, access to institutions and other aspects of their power. Whereas in the instance of disability the barriers to accessing assistance can be said to lie in the professional constructions of 'disability' in itself, in relation to refugees the barriers are more diffuse, in problems of cultural difference, the impact of trauma and also (perhaps more controversially) in debates about the legitimacy of any claims that they might make on the society of settlement.

A common thread in these two instances is that in both cases there is a problem of the balance between 'recognition' of disabled people or refugees as having reasonable claims on society and the way in which this affects 'redistribution' of the resources necessary for care and support to be achieved (compare with Hallahan 2015). There are key distinctions: in the first case, what it is to be a 'disabled person' has for so long been couched in terms of dependence, so that assertions of autonomy create the response of 'then why is assistance required?', while claims of a need for assistance in the case of refugees is met with the response of 'why is our community responsible for needs created somewhere else?' Nozick's (1974) argument that the misfortune of others is just bad luck and there is no injustice to be rectified also features in the underlying assumptions of some critics of social work and social welfare in these areas. Thus, in both areas the extent and shape of social welfare and the roles of social workers and others are highly contested.

Personal is (still) political: partnership, progress and social justice

We are faced now with a significant question: does Rawls's (1972) argument help us to consider social justice in social work and social welfare? To answer this, we need also to consider that in relation to the arguments of Rawls and Nozick there is also a third position, namely that Rawls does not go far enough. Whereas Rawls sees social justice in terms of equality of opportunity, others seek ways to ensure that this leads to demonstrable equality of outcomes. Feminist arguments, for example, have been used to question the apparent acceptance of various structural inequalities that the 'difference principle' can be used to support (for example, see Okin 1990). In other words, even accepting Rawls's basic notions in relation to issues of gender it is still possible to accept gender inequality.

From within social work, Solas (2008) and Banerjee (2011) have argued that Rawls's position is inadequate. Banerjee is particularly critical of two aspects of Rawls's ideas. First, he states that Rawls excludes health, including issues such as mental health and alcohol and other drug issues, from his conception of primary goods (those social goods that ought to be equitably distributed); second, it appears that Rawls ignores questions not only of gender but also of ethnic minorities, refugees and other marginal social groups. Moreover, Banerjee sees a significant shift in Rawls's thinking between 1972 and 2001, that Rawls reworked his original understanding to refocus from a moral conception of justice to a political one and in so doing to (re)introduce questions of desert into any considerations of the needs of those who are least well off (Rawls 2001). Solas advocates a more fundamental approach, asserting that radical egalitarianism should be the goal of social work and social welfare. In contrast, Banerjee is somewhat more qualified, but nevertheless also regards equality of outcome as the only acceptable measure of social justice.

It is not my purpose here to consider these differences, but rather to look at the broadly similar direction these critiques might take us. From these perspectives social work and social welfare ought to seek 'radical equality' and this involves politics as well as change at the level of individuals, families and communities. This would accord with Ife's (1997) position on the types of power that social workers ought to exercise within the social welfare field. In other words, social work and social welfare have a moral and political obligation, for Ife, only to engage with structural and community change that seeks to achieve social justice in the form of the greatest equality of outcome possible.

This seems to me to be both impractical and ethically questionable. The question of practicality is perhaps easier to identify. Even in the most consumer-controlled model of social welfare, there is a continuing need for professionals of various kinds to provide services or otherwise assist. While in many instances professional services and assistance may have been enacted in ways that are experienced as oppressive, there are forms of knowledge and skill that professionals gain through education and training that are not held by others. What is required to enable these to provide a means to pursue social justice is not that they are denied but that they are opened up to just social relations. This is seen not only in the necessity of professional power opened up at the level of changing policies, systems and structures (although that is a key part of what is necessary), but also that this is achieved at the level of individual human lives. Practical justice is achieved when for *this* person in *this* place at *this* time life is freer than before, not only when we can see an in-principle gain for communities or social classes. Yet lives can reasonably be different from each other and so a radical equality of outcome must, at the very least, be regarded in a very subtle and nuanced way. Freedom in this sense must be defined by the individuals, families and communities it concerns, above anyone else, otherwise we have simply replaced one professional dominance for another. In this respect some elements of Rawls's (1972) earlier formulation of the 'difference principle' still have something to offer.

Second, a practical objection to rejecting the micro (or individual) level of professional action reveals its ethical unacceptability. One of the most serious problems with the use of professional power in social welfare is that it is directed to rationing scarce resources. Of course, the world is finite. In recent times some critics have started to question whether expectations of social welfare do not also contribute to damage to the planet (Coates 2003). However, while accepting that the world is finite, the greatest reason for limiting the use of resources is that of intergenerational, environmental justice (Dominelli 2014, Besthorn *et al.* 2016). At the same time, any moral argument that supports the idea of social welfare has to find room for concepts of equality. That we might choose to limit present demands on the use of resources in order to ensure sufficient are available in the future for coming generations is a separate matter from how limited resources are distributed here and now. Yet the utilitarianism that has been the foundation of how access to social welfare has so often been structured, whether or not unwittingly, masks the way in which limitations have actually served the interest of greater accumulation of (material, cultural and social) goods by those who are most advantaged in society.

Some 25 years ago in an earlier discussion of power and caring, I considered the notion of 'democratic professionalism' (Hugman 1991). The ethical basis for this was to hold professions accountable to the foundational notion that, as Sercombe has since expressed it, '[we] do not provide a service we serve' (2010, p. 10). To create conditions of this type of democracy would require the reshaping of social relations between service users and professionals that market models have since been shown not to be able to sustain.

Banks (2012, pp. 93–94) has articulated a very clear framework for considering how social workers and other social welfare practitioners might build a socially just practice. The six elements to this that she proposes are as follows:

1   Making a thoroughgoing commitment to social justice a central value of theory and practice. This includes remaining critical of neo-liberal arguments that seek to confine questions of equity to 'equality of opportunity' and ignore issues of oppression.
2   Reframing empathy as the basis for social change and not only in order to focus on the needs of individuals. While individual lives matter, they must be seen in social context so that change occurs at all relevant levels.
3   Rethinking professional autonomy as 'relational autonomy', as well as the autonomy of service users (that has long been a goal of social work and social welfare). This again requires recognition that social context is important in defining and enabling autonomy.
4   Accepting collective responsibility for understanding and critiquing just and unjust conditions and practices. One example of how this can occur is when professional groups (such as associations) exercise power *with* service user groups.
5   Developing 'moral courage' to recognise and to challenge injustices in practices, systems and policies as well as seeking to protect the interests of the most vulnerable and disadvantaged members of a society.
6   Accepting that practices, systems and contexts are complex and contradictory. This may involve living with the difficulties of negotiating between the competing demands of the needs and interests of service users, policies, systems and wider social debates.

To these concepts I also want to add the notion of 'humility' (Hugman 2013, p. 89). By this I mean an acceptance that although professionals do have knowledge and skills that others do not, other forms of knowledge and skill are also valuable and should be respected in a practical relationship of power 'with' rather than 'over and above'. For example, in the mental health field the concepts of 'knowing from education' and 'knowing from experience' (as well as 'knowing by association') helps to understand that each participant in the interactions between professionals, service users and their families brings something to a relational process (Bland *et al.* 2015). Building just practice should incorporate this insight as foundational. Just action cannot be fully developed without just relationships or separately from just systems.

Plato's understanding of justice did not separate individuals from their social context: justice is *both* personal *and* political (Hinman 2013); nor should social work and social welfare in the early twenty-first century ignore this necessary connection. The practices and theories of social work were developed in contentious circumstances. That is, in the late nineteenth and early twentieth centuries they were highly and overtly political. In considering practical justice as just practice we have to recognise that this is still the case. So, social workers and social welfare practitioners must be prepared to contest the value of social justice as we seek to address poverty, disadvantage, marginalisation and other forms of social misery in the contemporary era.

Note

1 Drawing on the arguments of the Brandt Commission (1980), the term 'global North' as used in this chapter is roughly equivalent to the OECD members, and 'global South' for developing regions – see Hugman (2010) for further discussion.

References

Alston, M., 2009. *Innovative Human Services Practices: Australia's Changing Landscape.* South Yarra: Palgrave Macmillan.

Australian Association of Social Workers (AASW), 2010. *Code of Ethics.* Canberra: AASW.

Banerjee, M. M., 2011. Social Work Scholars' Representations of Rawls: A Critique. *Journal of Social Work Education*, 47 (2), 189–211.

Banks, S., 2004. *Ethics, Accountability and the Social Professions.* Basingstoke: Palgrave Macmillan.

Banks, S., 2012. *Ethics and Values in Social Work.* 4th edition. Basingstoke: Palgrave Macmillan.

Besthorn, F. H., Koenig, T. L., Spano, R. and Warren, S. L., 2016. A Critical Analysis of Social and Environmental Justice: Reorienting Social Work to an Ethic of Ecological Justice. In: R. Hugman and J. Carter, eds, *Rethinking Values and Ethics in Social Work.* London: Palgrave, 146–163.

Bland, R., Renouf, N. and Tullgren, A., 2015. *Social Work Practice in Mental Health.* 2nd edition. Sydney: Allen & Unwin.

Brandt Commission [The Independent Commission on International Development], 1980. *North-South: A Program for Survival.* London: Pan Books.

Castles, F. G., 1994. The Wage Earner's Welfare State Revisited. *Australian Journal of Social Issues,* 29 (2), 120–145.

Coates, J., 2003. *Ecology and Social Work: Towards a New Paradigm.* Halifax: Fernwood Press.

Dominelli, L., 2012. *Green Social Work: From Environmental Crisis to Environmental Justice.* Bristol: Polity Press.

England, H., 1983. *Social Work as Art.* London: George Allen & Unwin.

Esping-Andersen, G., 1990. *The Three Worlds of Welfare Capitalism.* Princeton, NJ: Princeton University Press.

Ferguson, I., 2008. *Reclaiming Social Work: Challenging Neo-liberalism and Promoting Social Justice.* London: Sage Publishers.

Gardner, F., 2014. *Practising Critical Reflection.* Basingstoke: Palgrave Macmillan.

Hallahan, L., 2015. Disability Policy in Australia: A Triumph of the *Scriptio Inferior* on Impotence and Neediness? *Australian Journal of Social Issues,* 50 (2), 191–208.

Healy, L. M., 2008. *International Social Work: Professional Action in an Interdependent World.* 2nd edition. New York: Oxford.

Hinman, L. M., 2013. *Ethics: A Pluralistic Approach to Moral Theory.* 5th edition. Boston, MA: Wadsworth.

Hugman, R., 1991. *Power in Caring Professions.* London: Macmillan.

Hugman, R., 1998. *Social Welfare and Social Value.* Basingstoke: Macmillan.

Hugman, R., 2010. *Understanding International Social Work: A Critical Analysis.* Basingstoke: Palgrave Macmillan.

Hugman, R., 2013. *Culture, Values and Ethics in Social Work: Embracing Diversity.* London: Routledge.

Ife, J., 1997. *Rethinking Social Work: Towards Critical Practice.* South Melbourne: Longman.

International Federation of Social Workers/International Association of Schools of Social Work (IFSW/IASSW), 2004. *Ethics in Social Work: Statement of Principles* [online]. Available from: http://ifsw.org/policies/statement-of-ethical-principles/ [Accessed 25 August 2016].

Locke, J., 1980 [1690]. *The Second Treatise on Government.* Ed. C. B. McPherson. Cambridge: Hackett Publishing Company.

Lymbery, M., 2014. Social Work and Personalisation: Fracturing the Bureau-Professional Compact? *British Journal of Social Work,* 44 (4), 795–811.

Nozick, R., 1974. *Anarchy, State and Utopia.* New York: Basic Books.

Okin, S. M., 1990. *Justice, Gender and the Family.* New York: Basic Books.

Oliver, M., Sapey, B. and Thomas, P., 2012. *Social Work with Disabled People.* 4th edition. Basingstoke: Palgrave Macmillan.

Osei-Hwedie, K., 1993. The Challenge of Social Work in Africa: Starting the Indigenisation Process. *Journal of Social Development in Africa,* 8 (1), 19–30.

Payne, M., 2005. *The Origins of Social Work.* Basingstoke: Palgrave Macmillan.

Postle, K. and Beresford, P., 2007. Capacity Building and the Reconception of Political Participation: A Role for Social Care Workers? *British Journal of Social Work,* 37 (1), 143–158.

Rawls, J., 1972. *A Theory of Justice*. Oxford: Clarendon Press.

Rawls, J., 2001. *Justice as Fairness: A Restatement*. Cambridge, MA: Belknap Press.

Robinson, K., 2014. Voices from the Front Line: Social Work with Refugees and Asylum Seekers in Australia and the UK. *British Journal of Social Work*, 44 (6), 1602–1620.

Seibel, F. W., ed., 2008. *Global Leaders for Social Work Education*. Ostrava: Verlag Albert/IASSW.

Sercombe, H., 2010. *Youth Work Ethics*. London: Sage Publications.

Singer, P., 2004. *One World: The Ethics of Globalization*. 2nd edition. New Haven, CT: Yale University Press.

Solas, J., 2008. Social Work and Social Justice – What are We Fighting for? *Australian Social Work*, 61 (2), 124–136.

Spicker, P., 1988. *Principles of Social Welfare*. London: Routledge.

Westoby, P., 2009. Developing a Community Development Approach through Engaging Resettling Southern Sudanese Refugees within Australia. *Community Development Journal*, 43 (4), 483–495.

Chapter 9

A just child protection system – is it possible?

Ilan Katz

Introduction

Ever since comprehensive systems have been implemented to protect children from maltreatment, debate has raged about the nature of those systems and how they can operate in a just manner. On the one hand, child protection systems exemplify the willingness of states to protect their most vulnerable citizens and therefore represent one of the crowning achievements of welfare states. On the other hand, these systems demonstrate the power of the state to enter into the lives of families, to override the authority of parents and carers and ultimately to break up family life.

This tension should not necessarily challenge the justice of the system. After all, everyone agrees that the system should protect 'the best interests of the child'. Therefore, in principle, everyone should have the same objectives: to protect children whose parents are unable or unwilling to provide them with adequate care, and to allow the rest of the population to get on with their family lives without the interference of the state. So why is there a problem for practical justice within child protection? Why is child protection policy characterised by tension, risk-aversion and constant debate about the most appropriate way forward? It turns out that 'the best interests of the child' is difficult to define and operationalise.

Child protection system challenges

Empirical evidence indicates a fundamental paradox in the way child maltreatment is managed in developed countries. Prevalence studies typically find that around 25 per cent of child maltreatment is never disclosed to authorities (Mathews *et al.* 2016). Yet child protection systems are inundated with reports, of which under 30 per cent are substantiated (AIHW 2017).[1]

This ever-increasing reporting activity places significant strain on the systems. Media attention has been a fundamental – and largely destructive – feature of child protection system reform over the past 50 years (Lonne *et al.* 2007). Indeed in the UK, for example, the system was first developed in response to a media scandal – namely, the death of Maria Caldwell in 1975. Since then, there have been countless scandals in which horrific child deaths are picked up by the media and the child protection system blamed for not preventing the death. This media attention has often led to commissions of inquiry, in many cases initiated by governments so that they can be shown to be 'doing something' about child abuse. These inquiries inevitably recommend the tightening of rules and procedures in order to prevent further deaths or serious abuse. This has in turn led to increasing bureaucratic and risk-averse practices, with the system being primarily geared towards avoiding media scrutiny and blame. The ultimate consequence of this cycle has been that, over time, more and more vulnerable families become entangled with the child protection system. Child protection systems are also criticised for being overzealous and for removing children from innocent parents who are merely trying to do their best. Again these cases are sensationalised in the media and practitioners blamed for breaking up loving families, leading to the 'damned if you do, damned if you don't' perception of the child protection system (Lonne *et al.* 2007).

These tensions have led to child protection systems being described as being 'in crisis' for about three decades (Parton 1991, Melton and Barry 1994). Multiple attempts at fundamental reform have been attempted in every jurisdiction in Australia and internationally.

Even more concerning is the fact that children report that child protection system intervention can be worse than the abuse itself. There are other injustices which seem to be inherent in the way child protection systems are configured. For example, in every country, minority and Indigenous children are over-represented in the child protection system (Katz and Connolly 2017). Another concern relates to children exposed to domestic and family violence. Exposure to violence in the family, even if the child is not physically abused, is now known to be highly damaging to children and is increasingly considered to be a form of maltreatment. Yet invoking the child protection system in cases of exposure to domestic and family violence can have detrimental effects on the children and their protective carers (usually the mothers) (Humphreys and Healy 2017). These issues will be explored in more depth below.

Although there is universal consensus about the ultimate aims of protecting children from harm, the child protection system faces significant challenges in achieving justice. Despite nearly 50 years of research and endless rounds of policy reform, the basic injustices of the child protection system persist. This raises the question – is a just child protection system possible?

Conceptions of child protection

Since the early 1990s, there have been constant debates about the fundamental orientation of the child protection system. Two basic models have been put forward in the literature, which are based on different views about the nature of child abuse and therefore the ultimate purpose of the child protection system. Comparative studies began in the 1990s, such as those of Gilbert (1997) and Cooper *et al.* (1995, 1997). These studies divided child protection systems into 'child protection' and 'family service' orientations. Broadly speaking, 'child protection' orientation is characteristic of English-speaking countries – the USA, the UK, Australia, New Zealand, Ireland and Canada, while continental European countries are characterised by having 'family service' orientations. Table 9.1, adapted from Gilbert (1997), summarises the difference between these two orientations. It is clear from this analysis that Gilbert (like most other commentators) was critical of the child protection orientation, because its basic premise is punitive and forensic, viewing parents who abuse their children essentially as culpable, whereas the family service model has a therapeutic orientation which understands abusive parents as fundamentally well intentioned but lacking appropriate skills and/or resources to address the needs of their children.

Underpinning these orientations are two fundamentally different conceptions of the nature of child abuse, and also of the role of the state. With regard to the role of the state, there is an interesting contradiction. Child protection oriented systems are characterised as being 'residual' in nature, with the state only intervening in cases of significant harm. However, the state is rather heavy handed, intervening in family life through intrusive investigations and assessments. In contrast, in family support systems the state is even more active, engaging with parents in support programmes even when there is no evidence of abuse. Although practitioners use statutory powers much more sparingly, they invoke the authority of the state to persuade families to engage with parenting programmes and other interventions. Both types of orientations therefore involve state intervention, but the intention and reception of the intervention differs between the risk-reduction interventions of child protection and the therapeutic interventions within family support.

In order to examine the implications of this for practical justice, it is useful to go beyond the systemic categorisation of these orientations and to

Table 9.1 Child protection and family service orientations

Child protection	Family service
Residual	Supportive
Forensic	Holistic
Investigation/assessment	Early intervention/support
Child-focused	Family-focused
Dualistic	Multi-dimensional

Source: adapted by the author from Gilbert (1997).

further examine the paradigms that underpin these two orientations: 'rescue' and 'public health'. These paradigms not only articulate deeper cultural understandings but also the appropriate response to child abuse. They represent two different conceptions of the nature of child abuse itself.

In the rescue paradigm child abuse is constructed as a crime. Thus the child protection system has an analogous function to the justice/police system: identifying and punishing perpetrators, supporting victims, and so on. Like the justice system, it is concerned with evidence and building a case against the perpetrator. In particular, the focus is on whether a crime has or has not been committed. If there is sufficient evidence that child abuse has occurred, perpetrators must pay the consequences.

In contrast, the public health paradigm, consistent with its name, views child abuse as a form of social 'disease'. In this conception, the child protection system is more analogous to a health system than a justice system. The primary modes of the health system are diagnosis and treatment, and investigations are aimed at gathering information which will be used to treat the 'patient' (parents). Public health is not focused on whether individuals do or do not have a particular disease. Rather, these systems are more holistically concerned about issues such as needs and lifestyles within the general population and/or vulnerable populations.

Child protection as rescue

Most child protection systems, particularly in English-speaking countries, were developed according to the rescue paradigm. The rescue trope is deeply embedded in our culture and is the topic of many fairy tales and myths as well as media reports and other narratives. Rescue involves three main actors – the hero/rescuer, the victim and the perpetrator. In the archetype, the victim is passive and must rely on the rescuer to be saved from the perpetrator by the hero. The appropriate response to these rescue situations are: pity for the victim, anger towards the perpetrator and gratitude towards the rescuer. The role of the rescuer is to save the victim from the perpetrator and the appropriate response for heroes is anger towards the perpetrator and pity for the victim. The appropriate response from the perpetrator are fear of the hero and shame towards the victim. This is a deep cultural trope and it is very difficult for individuals to step out of role, no matter what the specific circumstances of the case. The problem with this paradigm is that, when the script is not followed, the moral outrage and sense of injustice can shift, with unintended consequences. Thus in the scandals described above, the 'hero' fails to rescue the victim and thus public outrage becomes focused on the failures of the child protection system rather than the harm suffered by the child. Similarly, if the perpetrator is seen as innocent, the hero is perceived as being self-seeking and heavy-handed, wilfully removing children from loving and caring families.

It is now acknowledged that this model, while deeply culturally embedded and also offering the illusion of equity and accountability through extensive use of regulation and procedures, is fundamentally flawed. Research has shown that the victims of abuse are often as traumatised by the investigation and court processes as by the abuse itself (Plotnikoff and Woolfson 2005, Katz *et al.* 2017). Perhaps even more concerning, children who are removed from their parents and placed in out-of-home care appear to do no better, or even worse, than similar children who remain with their abusive parents (Doyle 2007). Overall, then, this model, while offering the appearance of justice, turns out to be unjust to parents, children, workers and the public.

Child protection as public health

The public health model of child protection was first proposed in Australia by Dorothy Scott, who strongly advocated a change of policy from the child protection orientation towards a public health model (Scott 2006). The public health model is the corollary of the view of child abuse as a disease. Like efforts in previous centuries to eliminate diseases such as cholera and typhoid, the public health model views the primary role of the child protection system as being to prevent the occurrence of the 'disease' and to treat those who succumb to it. Assessments of individual cases are therefore analogous to medical diagnosis rather than investigations of crime, and treatment of families is the appropriate response rather than punishment.

Importantly, those who have a disease are not generally considered personally responsible, and diseases result mainly from environmental and social factors, although personal behaviour does play some role in the public health response to conditions such as diabetes and obesity. The cultural response to public health issues is therefore somewhat ambivalent, focusing mainly on addressing social and environmental issues, but also containing an element of behaviour change. Nevertheless, public health is not concerned with punishment or retribution.

While appearing to be more just than the child protection model, the public health model has its own faults. Some of these are the converse of the child protection orientation. In particular, this model fails to deal with child abuse that is perpetrated by people (parents or others) who genuinely wish to harm children, rather than people who are unable to care for children adequately because they lack the resources or capacities to do so. In addition, some commentators (e.g. Featherstone *et al.* 2014) have challenged the concept of 'early intervention' in child protection, because it involves surveillance of vulnerable populations and unwarranted state interference in their lives on the basis that they are at high risk of abusing their children. While this conception of early intervention has been challenged by some (e.g. Axford and Berry 2018), even they acknowledge that the concept of early intervention has been used from time to time in policy to identify 'troubled' or 'at risk' families' (Ribbens McCarthy and Gillies 2018) and intervene in their lives, potentially resulting in stigmatisation and distress.

Child protection system reform

Neither the rescue nor public health models of child protection have been particularly successful (Gilbert *et al.* 2012, Russell *et al.* 2018). The rescue model, in particular, has been criticised, as indicated above, both for over-intrusiveness and also for a failure to protect children. The public health model is relatively successful for abuse which arises from family dysfunction, but struggles to deal with more serious types of abuse, in particular abuse which is closer to criminal behaviour, such as institutional abuse, cyber-abuse and trafficking. It also fails to address the concerns of victims of these types of abuse, many of whom wish for redress for themselves and punishment of offenders, rather than therapy or treatment (Katz *et al.* 2017).

More recent reform efforts have therefore attempted to combine these two perspectives, most recently by developing systems of 'differential response'. In these systems, reports are assessed and families are diverted either to the child protection or family support tracks, depending on the level of risk to the child and the needs of the family. To date, there is still ongoing debate about the effectiveness of this approach (Hughes *et al.* 2013, Merkel-Holguin and Bross 2015) and it is in any case a rather marginal solution – it does not deal with the underlying forensic and punitive nature of the process, nor the inequities which are built into the rescue model. One of the ironies of the current child protection or rescue systems is that there are increasing calls for reforms of the systems to make them more 'child centred' or 'child focused'. This is because most of the work undertaken within the systems is with adults. As victims, children have little say into how they will be protected, and their wider needs are often ignored.

Alternative conceptualisation of the child protection system

Both the crime and disease paradigms of child abuse, and their corollaries, the rescue and public health orientations, are, therefore, inadequate to the task of producing a system that offers justice to children, families and the community. Neither of these orientations acknowledge the complexity of the system, or the range of competing interests involved in protecting children and safeguarding their wellbeing. Although all systems on the continuum between rescue and public health models would claim to be protecting the 'best interests' of the child, the reality is that children's best interests are not the only driving force for any system, and, inevitably, other interests must be taken into account in developing a just system. Any system must take into account a range of competing interests and considerations in its development. Other than the best interest of the child, the system must provide justice to the child's family and community, to the workers in the system and to the public interest. This includes not only the public's confidence in the system but also the interests of the taxpayer and politicians. Of course, in an ideal world, these interests would all coincide with each other, and in some societies, at some times, all or most of these interests do cohere. For example, in Gilbert's original comparative research, and research by Cooper, Hetherington and colleagues in the 1990s, (Hetherington *et al.* 2001, Cooper *et al.* 2003) showed that in Europe, and particularly in Nordic countries, most, if not all of these interests did cohere at that time. These societies were all relatively socially and culturally homogenous, with a strong belief in the role of the state and its effectiveness to help and support families in need. The system was well resourced and was supported politically and socially. These conditions provided the context for a system which was accepted by the population at large as well as clients and workers within the system. More recent research shows that as these societies have become more diverse, and have moved towards neo-liberal service delivery models, the tensions in their child protection systems have increased considerably (Hennum 2017, Tham 2018).

The example of the Nordic countries indicates that the range of interests involved in the system will inevitably change as systems develop and as the contexts change. In the case of child protection, these contextual changes include technological changes (such as the Internet and online abuse), demographic developments (new immigrant groups within society, changing family structures), changes in societal norms (e.g. exposure to domestic and family violence being recognised as a child protection issue), broader legal and policy developments (criminal sanctions for sexual abuse increasing), economic changes and evidence from research and evaluation. Therefore, systems are in a constant state of evolution and development, although they tend to maintain their core values and orientations over long periods.

Disproportionality

One of the key injustices is the disproportionate number of minority ethnic and Indigenous children who have contact with the child protection system. This is an international phenomenon and is an ongoing characteristic of every child protection system across the globe. In fact, disproportionality is not only a feature of child protection; over-representation of clients from some minority communities is embedded into every human service system, particularly those which are more intrusive and punitive (Cunneen 2006). Although this is an international phenomenon, disproportionality is significantly greater in Australia than in most countries. In the USA and the UK, black and minority ethnic children are over-represented by a factor of around 2:1 (Putnam-Hornstein *et al.* 2013, Bywaters *et al.* 2016a, 2016b), whereas in Australia Aboriginal and Torres Strait Islander children are over-represented by a factor of 10:1 in the proportion of children in out-of-home care (AIHW 2017). Importantly, not all Indigenous and minority communities are over-represented in the child protection system. Some groups, such as Chinese and South Asian children, are under-represented, even when their socioeconomic circumstances are taken into account (Sawrikar and Katz 2013). This has implications for the credibility of some of the explanations for disproportionality. Although there is almost universal consensus that disproportionality is unjust,[2] there is considerable disagreement and debate about the causes of the injustice and the implications for both policy and practice. Furthermore, the disproportionality debate around child protection rests on certain assumptions which feed into larger debates in Australia about the appropriateness of policies and research relating to Aboriginal and Torres Strait Islander peoples. In particular is the assumption of 'white normality' – that is, that the proportion of children in the white (mainstream) population who are reported to the child protection system and are taken into care represents the benchmark against which other groups should be measured. The assumption here is that the average for the white population is the 'right' proportion, and that the extent to which children from Aboriginal and Torres Strait Islander communities differ from this benchmark represents the policy problem. However, in child protection, this is a totally arbitrary benchmark. As indicated in the introduction to this chapter, much child abuse is never reported to the child protection system, but also the child protection system is overwhelmed with reports and is making strenuous efforts to bring these numbers down. The proportion of children reported (or taken into care) indicates more about the system than about the problem in the community. There is in fact no 'right' number of children who should be reported or taken into care.

The assumption that the average for 'white Australia' should be the benchmark against which the Aboriginal and Torres Strait Islander community should be compared has been heavily criticised by many scholars in relation to the *Closing the Gap*[3] agenda, which similarly sets the white population averages as the benchmark for a range of outcomes which Indigenous peoples are expected to achieve (Kukutaia and Walter 2015). Even the basic language of 'disproportionality' and 'over-representation' is therefore laden with cultural assumptions about what is 'normal' and what is 'just', implicitly marginalising the experiences of Indigenous communities by viewing them only in comparison with the non-Indigenous experience. An alternative approach would be to engage in this debate by examining the concerns and experiences of Indigenous families who have been in contact with the child protection system and/or had their children removed and to develop policies and practices which meet the needs of those families.

The reasons for disproportionality in the child protection system have been extensively examined, but they signal two opposing theses; the first is that the child protection system itself is a racist institution which discriminates against Indigenous and minority communities. Discrimination is both a factor of conscious and unconscious prejudice and cultural insensitivity of individual workers in the system and/or institutional discrimination arising from policies and programmes. The alternative view is that the child protection system is not itself discriminatory. Rather, it is responding to higher prevalence of abuse and neglect in Indigenous communities, which is caused by intergenerational trauma due to colonialism, poverty, discrimination and lack of adequate services. Within these two opposing views are a number of assumptions and theoretical debates as well as empirical evidence. To date, there is no definitive answer to the issue, and it is probably the case that both these stances are true to some extent. The issues are explored in more depth in Katz and Connolly (2017). Here I will pick up a couple of concerns that are directly relevant to the question of justice in the child protection system.

One important question revolves around cultural competence, and in particular whether Aboriginal styles of parenting are misinterpreted by child protection workers as being neglectful or abusive, whereas they are culturally appropriate ways of parenting which are actually beneficial for the child in the context of Aboriginal society. Specifically, traditional Aboriginal methods of parenting are collective, whereby the biological mother of the child is only one of a range of carers. Children may spend time in various households and may often move around between households. Also, children are not punished for disobedience but are given role models for good behaviour and also given responsibilities in the community at a young age. This method of parenting is in tension with the concept of 'secure attachment' which underpins the theoretical basis of Western child development and child welfare practice. Those who accuse the child protection system of discrimination assert that culturally incompetent workers often remove Indigenous children because they are unaware of or insensitive to these differing patterns of parenting. The contrasting view is that traditional parenting styles were appropriate for the context of pre-colonial Indigenous societies, but are not appropriate in contemporary Western contexts, and are potentially neglectful. The empirical evidence indicates that, as in mainstream society, there are a very wide range of parenting practices amongst Indigenous families, and also that the traditional methods of parenting are beneficial for children (Lohoar *et al.* 2014). However, the extent to which non-Western parenting styles are a cause of the over-representation of Indigenous children being removed is not known.

Another issue relates to the tension between individual and collective justice. The child protection system is based on the notion of the 'best interests of the child'. As indicated above, this is a contested concept. For more than 40 years, the notion of 'best interests of the child' has been in widespread usage as a yardstick for guiding policy and practice in child care and protection. This is a basic concept embedded in the United Nations Convention on the Rights of the Child (UNCRC) (United Nations 1989). Nevertheless, as indicated above, there remain significant questions regarding the definition; 'best interests' of children are, or should be, defined in different cultural contexts and in particular the specific cultural views and understandings of children's interests (Alston and Gilmour-Walsh 1996, Leinaweaver 2014). Efforts to interpret and implement the Convention have encountered value conflicts across cultures and resistances at the local level (Harris-Short 2003).

The conflict is partly because the UNCRC is underpinned by notions of children's needs derived from 'Western' or 'global North' cultures (Holzscheiter 2010, Tisdall and Punch 2012) and it does not adequately take into account the wide differences in different cultural contexts relating to how children's wellbeing links to extended family and community (Walton 1976).

One of the key issues is the difference between individualist and collectivist cultures and how the different cultures address children's rights (Sawrikar and Katz 2017). As indicated in the discussion on the 'rescue' model, child protection systems are underpinned by a fundamentally individual concept of the best interests of the child, in which the immediate protection of the child is paramount. On the one hand, this model can support victims of abuse who are pressurised not to disclose in order to maintain the 'face' or reputation of the community. Protection, and especially removal, of children can nevertheless have significant negative consequences for communities as well as individual children. In the case of Aboriginal and Torres Strait Islanders, this is most dramatically evidenced in the Stolen Generations[4] policies, which were damaging to both the children concerned and their communities collectively (HREOC 1997). However, even when it is in each child's best interests to be removed from the family, the collective impact of such removals or interventions on communities can be extremely damaging. The ongoing high level of removals of Indigenous children in Australia and other countries is viewed by those communities as a continuation of colonialist policies which ultimately destroy intergenerational continuity and the integrity of the community. Similarly, it has been argued that inter-country adoption is a manifestation of neo-colonialism, with rich countries benefiting from the misfortune of parents in developing countries who are not able to provide for their children. Thus, even if the individual children benefit from being internationally adopted, the institution of inter-country adoption replicates the colonial enterprise, removing resources from poor countries in order to satisfy the needs of people in rich countries (Efrat *et al.* 2015).

Conclusion

These two examples, concerning how differences in parenting are interpreted and the tension between individual and community rights, indicate the complexity for policymakers and practitioners aiming to move towards a more just child protection system.

They show how the basic concepts such as 'best interests', 'safety' and 'need' become problematic when applied in different cultural and social contexts. Ultimately the child protection system is part of mainstream society and so the question 'is the child protection system racist or is disproportionality a factor of the broader society?' is not by itself the most meaningful. The child protection system was designed within the cultural constraints of a society in which the individualist rescue model is so embedded that it is considered to be culturally neutral. Therefore, disproportionality is likely to be embedded in the basic design of the system, rather than being caused by individual practitioners' and managers' conscious or unconscious racist stereotypes. Reforms which move the system towards a public health model or a differential response approach are likely to have limited impact on this factor. The child protection system is likely to remain controversial and contested, continuing to have to juggle the interests and safety of children against those of parents, communities and other stakeholder groups.

In particular, the global struggle for justice within the child protection systems for children from Indigenous and minority ethnic communities still has a long way to go. Although there is now much more understanding of the dynamics of over- and under-representation in the child protection system, there is ongoing and vigorous debate about how these issues could be resolved. Unfortunately, the system is driven by a number of factors which undermine the search for justice. These include the risk-averse nature of public services and in particular child protection, cowardly political leadership which prefers to blame practitioners and managers rather than its own policies, lack of funding and the pursuit of 'quick fixes' such as expensive 'evidence based' programmes which are 'guaranteed' to improve outcomes.

Fundamental reform of the system has been illusory and is unlikely to be achieved within the current policy and cultural settings. Child protection is couched within a network of other human services which similarly have to balance different interests. Continuous reform is therefore likely to be a feature for the long term and it is important to believe that the system can somehow 'muddle through'. A system that provides justice to all stakeholders is not possible, but one that effectively balances the competing interests of different groups is potentially achievable, although it is unlikely that any of the stakeholder groups will readily recognise it as such.

Notes

1 In 2015–16, there were 162,175 children receiving child protection services in Australia, of whom 45,714 were subjects of substantiations.
2 This is not quite true; some right-wing commentators such as Sammut (2015) have called for more Indigenous and non-Indigenous children to be removed from their families and adopted. This is also a view taken by some of the right-wing media.
3 *Closing the Gap* is the Australian Government's commitment to address disparities between Aboriginal and Torres Strait Islander people and mainstream Australia. The policy was announced by Prime Minister Kevin Rudd in 2008. Each year a report is presented to parliament showing progress against seven targets. See https://closingthegap.pmc.gov.au/.
4 The *Stolen Generations* refers to the policies of Australian governments in the nineteenth and twentieth centuries to remove Aboriginal and Torres Strait Islander children from their communities and place them in institutions or with white families in order to civilise them and integrate them into mainstream Australian society.

References

AIHW, 2017 *Child Protection Australia 2015–16.* Canberra: Australian Institute of Health and Welfare (AIHW).
Alston, P. and Gilmour-Walsh, B. 1996. *The Best Interests of the Child: Towards a Synthesis of Children's Rights and Cultural Values.* Florence: UNICEF International Child Development Centre.
Axford, N. and Berry, V., 2018. Perfect Bedfellows: Why Early Intervention Can Play a Critical Role in Protecting Children – A Response to Featherstone *et al.* (2014) 'A Marriage Made in Hell: Child Protection Meets Early Intervention'. *British Journal of Social Work*, 48 (1), 254–273. doi: 10.1093/bjsw/bcx003.
Bywaters, P., Brady, G., Sparks, T. and Bos, E., 2016a. Child Welfare Inequalities: New Evidence, Further Questions. *Child & Family Social Work*, 21, 369–380. doi: 10.1111/cfs.12154.
Bywaters, P., Brady, G., Sparks, T. and Bos, E., 2016b. Inequalities in Child Welfare Intervention Rates: The Intersection of Deprivation and Identity. *Child & Family Social Work*, 21, 452–463. doi: 10.1111/cfs.12161.
Cooper, A., Hetherington, R., Baistow, K., Pitts, J. and Spriggs, A., 1995. *Positive Child Protection: A View from Abroad.* Lyme Regis: Russell House Publishing.
Cooper, A., Hetherington, R. and Katz, I., 1997. *The Third Way: A European Perspective of the Child Protection/Family Support Debate.* London: NSPCC.

Cooper, A., Hetherington, R. and Katz, I., 2003. *The Risk Factor: Making the Child Protection System Work for Children.* London: Demos.

Cunneen, C., 2006. Racism, Discrimination and the Over-Representation of Indigenous People in the Criminal Justice System: Some Conceptual and Explanatory Issues. *Current Issues in Criminal Justice,* 17 (3), 329–346.

Doyle, J. J., 2007. Child Protection and Child Outcomes: Measuring the Effects of Foster Care. *American Economic Review,* 97 (5), 1583–1610.

Efrat, A., Leblang, D., Liao, S. and Pandya, S. S., 2015. Babies across Borders: The Political Economy of International Child Adoption. *International Studies Quarterly,* 59, 615–628.

Featherstone, B., Morris, K. and White, S., 2014. A Marriage Made in Hell: Early Intervention Meets Child Protection. *British Journal of Social Work,* 44 (7), 1735–1749.

Gilbert, N., 1997. *Combatting Child Abuse: International Perspectives and Trends.* New York, Oxford: Oxford University Press.

Gilbert, R., Fluke, J., O'Donnell, M., Gonzalez-Izquierdo, A., Brownell, M., Gulliver, P., Janson, S. and Sidebotham, P., 2012. Child Maltreatment: Variation in Trends and Policies in Six Developed Countries. *Lancet,* 379, 758–772. doi: 10.1016/S0140-6736(11)61087-8.

Harris-Short, S., 2003. International Human Rights Law: Imperialist, Inept and Ineffective? Cultural Relativism and the UN Convention on the Rights of the Child. *Human Rights Quarterly,* 25 (1), 130–181.

Hennum, N., 2017. The Norwegian Child Protection Services in Stormy Weather. *Critical and Radical Social Work,* 5 (2), 1–15. doi: 10.1332/204986017X15029695863676.

Hetherington, R., Baistow, K., Trowell, J., Katz, I. and Mesie, J., 2001. *The Children of Parents with Mental Illness: Learning from Inter-country Comparisons.* Chichester: Wiley.

Holzscheiter, A., 2010. *Children's Rights in International Politics: The Transformative Power of Discourse.* New York: Palgrave Macmillan.

HREOC, 1997. *Bringing Them Home: Report of the National Inquiry into the Separation of Aboriginal and Torres Strait Islander Children from Their Families.* Canberra: Human Rights and Equal Opportunities Commission.

Hughes, R. C., Rycus, J. S., Saunders-Adams, S. M., Hughes, L. K. and Hughes, K. N., 2013. Issues in Differential Response. *Research on Social Work Practice,* 23 (5), 493–520. doi: 10.1177/1049731512466312.

Humphreys, C. and Healy, L., 2017. *Pathways and Research in Collaborative Interagency Practice: Collaborative Work across the Child Protection and Specialist Domestic and Family Violence Interface.* Sydney: Australia's National Research Organisation for Women's Safety (ANROWS).

Katz, I. and Connolly, M., 2017. Disproportionality and Risk Decision-making in Child Protection. In: M. Connolly, ed., *Beyond the Risk Paradigm in Child Protection: Current Debates and New Directions.* London: Palgrave, 63–76.

Katz, I., Jones, A., Newton, B. J. and Reimer, E., 2017. *Life Journeys of Victim/Survivors of Child Sexual Abuse in Institutions: An Analysis of Royal Commission Private Sessions for the Royal Commission into Institutional Responses to Child Sexual Abuse.* Sydney: Royal Commission into Institutional Responses to Child Sexual Abuse.

Kukutaia, T. and Walter, M., 2015. Recognition and Indigenizing Official Statistics: Reflections from Aotearoa New Zealand and Australia. *Statistical Journal of the IAOS,* 31 (6), 317–332. doi: 10.3233/SJI-150896.

Leinaweaver, J., 2014. Informal Kinship-based Fostering around the World: Anthropological Findings. *Child Development Perspectives*, 8 (3), 131–136. doi: 10.1111/cdep. 12075.

Lohoar, S., Butera, N. and Kennedy, E. 2014. *Strengths of Australian Aboriginal Cultural Practices in Family Life and Child Rearing: CFCA Paper No. 25*. Melbourne: Australian Institute of Family Studies.

Lonne, B., Parton, N., Thomson, J. and Harries, M., 2007. *Reforming Child Protection*. London: Routledge.

Mathews, B., Walsh, K., Dunne, M., Katz, I., Arney, F., Higgins, D., Octoman, O., Parkinson, S. and Bates, S., 2016. *Scoping Study for Research into the Prevalence of Child Abuse in Australia: Report to the Royal Commission into Institutional Responses to Child Sexual Abuse*. Sydney: Social Policy Research Centre, UNSW Australia in partnership with Australian Institute of Family Studies, Queensland University of Technology and the Australian Centre for Child Protection (University of South Australia).

Melton, G. B. and Barry, F. D., 1994. *Protecting Children from Abuse and Neglect: Foundations for a New National Strategy*. New York: Guilford Press.

Merkel-Holguin, L. and Bross, D. C., 2015. Commentary: Taking a Deep Breath before Reflecting on Differential Response. *Child Abuse & Neglect*, 39, 1–6. doi: http://dx.doi.org/10.1016/j.chiabu.2014.11.017.

Parton, N., 1991. *Governing the Family: Child Care, Child Protection and the State*. London: Macmillan Education.

Plotnikoff, J. and Woolfson, R., 2005. *In Their Own Words: The Experiences of 50 Young Witnesses in Criminal Proceedings*. London: NSPCC and Victim Support.

Putnam-Hornstein, E., Needell, B., King, B. and Johnson, M., 2013. Racial and Ethnic Disparities: A Population-based Examination of Risk Factors for Involvement with Child Protective Services. *Child Abuse & Neglect*, 37 (1), 33–46. doi: http://dx.doi.org/10.1016/j.chiabu.2012.08.005.

Ribbens McCarthy, J. and Gillies, V., 2018. Troubling Children's Families: Who's Troubled and Why? Approaches to Inter-cultural Dialogue. *Sociological Research Online*, 23 (1), 219–244. doi: 10.1177/1360780417746871.

Russell, J. R., Kerwin, C. and Halverson, J. L., 2018. Is Child Protective Services Effective? *Children and Youth Services Review*, 84, 185–192. doi: https://doi. org/10.1016/j.childyouth.2017.11.028.

Sammut, J., 2015. *The Madness of Australian Child Protection: Why Adoption Will Rescue Australia's Underclass Children*. Sydney: Connorcourt Publishing.

Sawrikar, P. and Katz, I., 2013. 'Normalizing the Novel': How Is Culture Addressed in Child Protection Work with Ethnic-minority Families in Australia? *Journal of Social Service Research*, 40 (1), 39–61. doi: 10.1080/01488376.2013.845126.

Sawrikar, P. and Katz, I., 2017. How Aware of Child Sexual Abuse (CSA) Are Ethnic Minority Communities? A Literature Review and Suggestions for Raising Awareness in Australia. *Children and Youth Services Review*, 81, 246–260. doi: https://doi.org/10.1016/j.childyouth.2017.08.015.

Scott, D. A., 2006. Towards a Public Health Model of Child Protection in Australia. *Communities, Families and Children Australia*, 1 (1), 9–16.

Tham, P., 2018. A Professional Role in Transition: Swedish Child Welfare Social Workers' Descriptions of Their Work in 2003 and 2014. *British Journal of Social Work*, 48 (1), 449–467.

Tisdall, E. K. M. and Punch, S., 2012. Not so 'New'? Looking Critically at Childhood Studies. *Children's Geographies*, 10 (3), 249–264. doi: 10.1080/14733285.2012.693376.

United Nations, 1989. *United Nations Convention on the Rights of the Child 1989*. Available from: www.ohchr.org/Documents/ProfessionalInterest/crc.pdf.

Walton, R., 1976. The Best Interests of the Child. *British Journal of Social Work*, 6 (3), 307. doi: 10.1093/oxfordjournals.bjsw.a056730.

Chapter 10

Collaborative disability-inclusive research and evaluation as a practical justice process

Karen R. Fisher and Rosemary Kayess

Introduction

Academia rarely moves aside to make room for inclusive practice in research and teaching, despite much rhetoric about social justice and equity. People with disabilities demand equality in education, yet remain under-represented as students, teachers and researchers on campus. One approach to correcting this injustice is to critically examine research practice and develop new structural and relational responses that demonstrate alternative methodologies. The research conducted by the authors in conjunction with university and community colleagues has engaged in that methodological struggle for several decades. This chapter explores how close collaboration with people with disabilities and the organisations that represent them is transforming research practice and, consequently, research impact. It uses examples of research projects initiated by community partners or government to illustrate how the approach changed the research questions that were asked, the methods that were applied and the way in which the results were used.

We begin by positioning the question of collaborative research practice as a practical justice process within the context of the UN Convention on the Rights of Persons with Disabilities 2008 (CRPD n.d.). We emphasise why and how rights to inclusive education and research are interrelated and the power structures that resist these changes. We argue that positioning collaborative research practice conducted within the normative rights framework of the CRPD can guide researchers towards a form of inclusive practice that is capable of generating transformative evidence, in ways not possible for academics or Disabled Persons Organisations working apart. We present two case studies in which collaborative processes were adopted to try to achieve greater inclusivity. Findings from these demonstrate how collaborative research can contribute to transformative practices in the community and impact on policy.

Right to participate in research about disability

Participation in disability research can usefully be understood within a rights framework. The CRPD seeks to bring about a paradigm shift in disability policy based on an understanding of people with disabilities as rights-holders and human rights subjects. Until relatively recently, public discourse and policy in the area of disability was commonly characterised as a deficit of the individual, rather than attributing the problem to the social attitudes and environment. This approach to disability as an individual deficiency reinforced notions of disability as difference or 'other'. In response, public policy focused on separate parallel institutions and services in isolation to mainstream systems (Kayess and Smith 2016). Separate education meant historically low levels of academic achievement, which kept people with disabilities out of key professions and public administration (Linton 1998). As a result, they have not been represented in public decision-making processes on law and policy. Disability has also been a marginalised area for academic research concern, which has led to limited understanding of the issues it raises.

In contrast, inclusion embraces human rights principles such as respect for human dignity by reflecting and celebrating human diversity. Degener (2016) argues the underlying equality concept of the CRPD can be categorised as transformative equality. This approach to equality requires the removal of barriers to inclusion and positive measures to accommodate difference and initiate structural change (Fredman 2011, p. 30).

As a transformative enabler, the CRPD provides a normative framework to build the capacity of states, aimed at addressing deficits of technical and bureaucratic capability and policy resources. Central to this is an informed policy evidence base that reflects the experience of people with disabilities. Disability advocates have long made claims for 'Nothing About Us, Without Us' (Charlton 1998) to participate in the policy process and have a voice in the policy discourse. This was a central demand of Disabled Persons Organisations during the CRPD negotiations. James Charlton used the phrase to challenge the powerlessness and oppression of people with disabilities in recognition of decades of public policy that failed to include people with disabilities and left them trapped in systems of care, treatment and protection. Charlton's words have come to represent a claim to rights and recognition following years of exclusion and social isolation and have been a driving force behind the transformative nature of the CRPD.

The CRPD as a transformative project is about addressing the failure of public policy to include the voices and experience of people with disability. The outcome of the prolonged UN negotiations between states, supported by non-states parties such as Disabled Persons Organisations, resulted in a normative framework that holds states accountable for their commitment to realise the rights of people with disabilities. Researchers and their partners now have the opportunity to use this public framework to pursue practical justice processes and goals in their research.

The CRPD incorporates several elements that foster capacity-building. Central to these mechanisms are research and development and ongoing engagement with persons with disability and their representative organisations. The CRPD also enshrines a right to inclusive lifelong educational opportunities. Education plays an important and interrelated role in facilitating the ability of people with disabilities to engage in the social discourse and inform the policy discourse. Education enables their participation in community life. Article 24 – Education in the CRPD provides that all people with disabilities have the right to education in an inclusive education system. This includes being able to access general tertiary education, vocational training and adult education on an equal basis with others.

Yet many people with disabilities experience greatly inferior education compared with their peers, often as a result of inadequate levels of disability support to accommodate their learning, with poor quality curricula and instructional methods greatly diminishing their academic development (Kayess forthcoming). World Health Organization (WHO)-sponsored research presents a global portrait of exclusion and obstructed capability. Across 51 countries participating in the World Health Survey (WHO 2011), people with disabilities experienced significantly lower rates of primary school completion and fewer years of education than those without disability. A similar portrait emerges from a survey of the Concluding Observations of the CRPD between 2011 and 2017 (CRPD n.d.). The overwhelming placement of people with disabilities in segregated schools and the lack of access to inclusive education are almost universal, even in high-income countries (CRPD n.d.). Exclusion from tertiary education is similar. OECD figures show people with disabilities experience significant barriers to, and have limited transition to, tertiary education (OECD 2011).

People with disabilities are disadvantaged in terms of their access to and participation in higher education in Australia. Similar to Europe, their share of enrolment is growing, but in the 15–65 years age group, only 15 per cent of people with disabilities have a bachelor's degree or higher, compared with 26 per cent of other people (Eurostat 2014). This lack of access to education and in particular higher education is reflected in the disproportionately low representation in key professions, which limits the voice of disability in social, policy and political discourse. Limited representation in academia further compounds the situation by disability not being considered an area of concern or limiting the lived experience of disability from informing the evidence base of policy development. Inclusive research is an avenue through which these limitations can be addressed.

The CRPD sets out obligations about research in Article 4 – General Obligations, which includes promoting research and development. It identifies engagement with people with disabilities as a central element in the implementation and monitoring of the human rights and fundamental freedoms contained in the Convention. The preambular paragraph (0) acknowledges that 'persons with disability should have the opportunity to be actively involved in decision making processes about policies and programmes, including those directly concerning them'. Article 31 – Statistics and Data Collection requires that countries collect information, including statistical and research data, to enable them to formulate and implement policies to give effect to the Convention, including addressing the barriers faced by persons with disabilities in exercising their rights. Article 33 embraces this active dialogue with persons with disability and their representative organisations. Engagement with people with disabilities is central to informed policy by promoting a greater understanding of the lived experience of disability. An understanding of the lived experience of disability is critical, not only in informing policy developments and law reform, but also in monitoring and highlighting human rights abuses (Kayess and Smith 2016). In total, these Articles require the inclusion of people with disabilities in research processes to effect their rights.

Collaborating in disability-inclusive research

Inclusive processes provide opportunities for people with disabilities to develop research skills and embeds the lived experience of disability in research methodology. Disability-inclusive research is an approach to research that can address inequities in research participation. It was developed in response to the exclusion of people with intellectual disability (Walmsley and Johnson 2003, Nind and Vinha 2014). In Australia, Ollerton and Horsfall (2013) demonstrated how the process of conducting inclusive participatory action research using a human rights framework with people with intellectual disability led to social change. Their project examined the group's experience of rights expressed in the CRPD, which resulted in them requesting that the academic researchers took actions to support them to demand local changes that would enable their rights.

Collaborative research is a general term adopted in evaluation and applied research to describe various forms of co-production, inclusive and participatory research (Cousins *et al.* 2016). These practices are particularly relevant where the research is formative or transformative in its aims and processes (Mertens 2009). Cousins *et al.* (2016) have developed over time a framework for understanding the goals, interests, processes and forms of collaborative critical inquiry. Their application is primarily to evaluation, although we would argue it is equally relevant to other types of applied research.

The Cousins *et al.* collaborative research framework includes three main features. The first of these focuses on what may be described as the antecedent conditions for the research, such as the alignment between stakeholders about information needs, understanding of the problem and what the research is intended to accomplish. Second, the framework considers the purpose of the research, which may include the overlapping justifications of the practical (problem-solving and instrumental use of evidence), the political (transformative in the interests of social inclusion and justice), and the philosophical (constructivist understanding of meanings and representations of policy experience). Third, the framework includes the forms of enquiry that typify different collaborative research approaches: control of technical decision-making in the research; diversity in the range of stakeholders engaged; and depth of participation in the methodological elements of the study.

Cousins *et al.* applied this framework to understand when collaborative research is more likely to be successful. They found that the critical factors were when there is a high level of stakeholder agreement about the needed information; when the expressed purpose of the research is to use it by learning from a thorough understanding of the programme; and when a wider range and deeper level of stakeholder participation is adopted in the collaboration. They noted that these findings are important where the aim of the research is transformative and practical because the research collaboration brings people and organisations together throughout the research process. Interestingly, control of technical decisions did not differentiate the successful projects, perhaps indicating a role for the academic researcher in a collaborative approach.

Participation in disability policy research provides a site for collaborative research to overcome the typically asymmetrical power relations between people with disabilities who are intended to benefit from the policies and other stakeholders, including government, service providers and academic researchers. The purpose of inclusive research processes in this context can be to influence policy and practice of governments and markets both through the research processes and the generation of relevant knowledge, a demonstration of all three of Cousins *et al.*'s justifications – practical, political and philosophical – which resonate strongly with the pursuit of practical justice.

Historically, under charity and welfare models of disability policy, people with disabilities were largely excluded or marginalised from the policy process. Unfortunately remnants of that approach still dominate in the way disability experiences are often framed in policy and research. Partly this is due to where and how research is initiated and funded, usually by government, service providers or academics, and less often by community groups or representative organisations. The type of research is often a policy or programme evaluation, which can limit the scope and resources for alternative methodologies. In addition, the content of disability policy research is often restricted to disability support rather than a broader focus on active citizenship.

In an attempt to remedy these tendencies, Robinson *et al.* (2014) applied an earlier version of Cousins *et al.*'s framework (Weaver and Cousins 2004) to identify the effectiveness of extending inclusive approaches to disability policy research. They found that although inclusive practices were feasible and changed the policy process, the depth of inclusivity and power shift within the research team towards people with disabilities required greater resource investment and commitment to build the capacity of people with disabilities, and to ensure their representative organisations and academics to work together in more equitable ways.

Here we apply Cousins *et al.*'s collaborative critical inquiry framework of antecedent conditions, the purpose of the research and the form of inquiry to understand how collaboration with people with disabilities and the organisations that represent them is transforming research practice and impact. The case studies that follow are analysed by describing the research project, analysing the research practice employed against Cousins *et al.*'s collaboration framework and examining the impact of the project on policy and practice.

Spinal Cord Injury Australia research

A research project with Spinal Cord Injury Australia (SCIA) provides a useful entry point to this discussion because of the way that it was commissioned, and the partnership between the organisation and university that conducted it. SCIA is a Disabled Persons Organisation governed by people with disabilities that supports people with spinal cord injury (SCI) and other similar disabilities to overcome barriers, achieve goals and live fulfilling lives (https://scia.org.au/).

The research project emerged from an existing organisational and professional relationship between SCIA managers and researchers in the Social Policy Research Centre at UNSW Sydney. Through several discussions, they prioritised research opportunities that would be most useful for the organisation's members. The discussions set out to define the purpose of the research that might address problems and barriers that members experienced. The design process identified so many problems that SCIA realised that it did not know the priority of questions, what the members were experiencing and what was holding them back. SCIA managers decided that a general research question for 'blue-skies' research into barriers to life choices was most suitable in these circumstances. The research aimed to examine the impact of spinal cord injury on people's life experiences and identified gaps and barriers to achieving self-fulfilment. The research, which was conducted with SCIA staff, included key informant roundtables, in-depth interviews with 15 people with a spinal cord injury and a survey of SCIA members. The SCIA later used the results of the research to set strategic directions that enable each person with a spinal cord injury to choose from a range of life choices (Bates *et al.* 2013).

The study design included mutual capacity-building of the research capacity of SCIA staff and the inclusive practice capacity of university research staff. It adopted an appreciative approach to enquiry (Rogers and Fraser 2003) to focus on the achievements of participants; a social inclusion framework for analysis for comparison with the rights of the wider population (learning, working, engaging and influencing; Australian Government 2012); and the Personal Wellbeing Index for a comparative quantitative benchmark to other Australian citizens. People with spinal cord injury were included in the research team, including Rosemary Kayess, the principal investigator and SCIA staff member. SCIA staff supported the project by participating in the design and analysis. The organisation's members participated in all the methods, including the interviews, survey and roundtables. The roundtables were to seek their input into the design and analysis of the data from the other sources. The outcomes from the research were presented to the SCIA management board, the majority of whom are people with disabilities. The SCIA used the research as the basis for their strategic planning to guide their priorities and work plan of the organisation. Through this process, the research raised the SCIA's profile as an organisation that focuses on the voices of people with spinal cord injury. As a membership organisation, it was important for the SCIA to represent its members and the research framed this in a way that policymakers understood and could apply.

In the Australian context, a major response to the CRPD has been the National Disability Insurance Scheme (NDIS), an approach to the individualised funding of disability supports. The NDIS is a core element of the Australian Government's National Disability Strategy, which is directed to meeting Australia's obligations under the CRPD. The scheme is a significant shift away from a welfare model in which people with disabilities had little choice and no certainty of access to appropriate supports. The NDIS embraces the human rights principles of the CRPD of making one's own choices. Designed to increase community participation, the NDIS provides people with disabilities the means to make choices about the goals in their lives and what supports they require to achieve them. The SCIA research's use of the social inclusion framework, methodology and research outcomes was compatible with these broader policy shifts. The report was launched at Parliament House in the Australian capital city, Canberra, by the relevant minister, with politicians from other parties, other service providers and community members. The profile of the research prompted responses from politicians, government and NGOs, such as invitations to be involved in other projects.

Crucially, this work provided the evidence base to support the advocacy work of the SCIA. It provided a rich demonstration of the organisation's capacity to pursue practical justice through collaborative research. The implications of the findings in the report were framed in terms of responsibilities of the SCIA, government and wider community. The SCIA took up an advocacy role for the latter two. It also armed the SCIA with evidence for proposals to government to financially support the SCIA's proposed directions. Because the proposed directions were derived from members' priorities, it was easier to justify them. Moreover, applying collaborative, inclusive research within this project meant that the research questions, methods, analysis and application turned out differently from what had been anticipated by either partner. For example, the SCIA initially came to the university researchers with a utilitarian question about housing, which changed to a broader more normative approach after the first roundtable participants insisted the framework should change to personal, family and community resources, based on their experiences.

My Choice Matters evaluation

The My Choice Matters evaluation offers a second case study because it provides an example of how to effectively manage the power relationships between a representative organisation, the government and the university. In this case, when the Disabled Persons Organisation, the NSW Council for Intellectual Disability (CID), was developing a competitive proposal to government for a capacity-building programme, they included the Social Policy Research Centre, UNSW Sydney as the evaluation partner, because of the prior history of successful research collaboration between the CID and the university. Previously, CID members and staff had participated in research led by the university as advisors, trainers or researchers. This, however, was the first study where work was led by the CID.

The university evaluated the process and impact of the programme as part of the CID's programme management obligations to the government funder. My Choice Matters supports people with disabilities and their families to increase their skills, knowledge and confidence in making choices and taking control of their lives, in particular self-directed support and individualised budgets. The programme prioritised inclusive practice in the way it was managed and conducted, for example, running workshops that were accessible to people who did not read. The evaluation analysed how the programme contributed to people's skills and knowledge; their capacity to take action; and the facilitators and barriers to successful outcomes. It used mixed methods, including focus groups, interviews, feedback forms and inclusive approaches to adapt these methods as required to include all people with disabilities involved in the programme (Meltzer *et al.* 2013).

In the study, people with disabilities led the evaluation and were part of the team for the research design. A community researcher with intellectual disability was employed to advise on the accessibility and content of research instruments, easy-read advice, and support and training for field-work team members. All the research materials were adapted to accessible formats. Members of the advisory group of the programme, who were people with disabilities and families, informed both the design of the programme and the evaluation methodology.

The evaluation was designed to include regular meetings with programme management for formative evaluation feedback so that findings from the early research waves could inform programme improvement. For example, the evaluation identified that engagement with more marginalised groups such as Indigenous people was not initially successful, so a more targeted approach was adopted in later implementation. In this way, the inclusive evaluation enabled reflective practice between the researchers and programme teams to identify and resolve implementation problems. In response, the CID designed new sessions to target specific community groups.

The evaluation findings provided an evidence base for the CID to identify new priority areas for capacity building, which they proposed to government (Griffiths *et al.* 2017). For example, the early waves of the evaluation identified that the way the programme was initially designed was unable to reach people living in formal residential care. The CID successfully sought a supplementary programme to reach into these settings. An interesting benefit of the collaboration was the way in which the inclusive practice of the researchers and the Disabled Persons Organisation challenged and influenced each other. For example, because the research team included people with disabilities, it identified gaps in the inclusivity of the programme that the Disabled Persons Organisation was able to address. Similarly, the Disabled Persons Organisation suggested inclusive ways of seeking evaluation feedback from workshop participants.

Implications of collaboration for practice justice

The chapter has addressed the question of how collaboration with people with disabilities and the organisations that represent them can transform research practice and impact. It has applied Cousins *et al.*'s collaborative critical inquiry framework, with its three dimensions of antecedent conditions; the purpose of the research; and the form of inquiry to examine two case studies where university researchers and Disabled Persons Organisations collaborated in research and evaluation projects. It has adopted a critical approach to examine how collaborative research can contribute to transformative policy and practice through practical, political and philosophical change. The case studies reveal that the two collaborations had transformative implications for some of the people, organisations and researchers involved, and changed the research processes and impact.

The antecedent conditions relevant to the success of the collaborations in the case studies were that the researchers and organisations had long-term relationships before the research projects were designed or commenced. This meant that they were in a position of mutual trust to explore new research questions, in the case of the SCIA, and new inclusive formative research methods, in the case of the CID. Their shared understanding of the research problems were assisted by the explicit social justice values base of the university researchers, as specialist disability policy researchers, including researchers with disabilities. This meant that the researchers and organisations were personally and institutionally aware of the contextual policy problems and context in which the research was conducted and what was intended to be accomplished. The collaborative research design process also contributed to reaching shared agreements on the research focus.

The focus of the research in both cases lent itself to collaborative inquiry for different reasons. In the SCIA research, the mutually derived design required deep involvement from SCIA staff and members to be successful. It would otherwise have been difficult to engender trust from participants to self-critically reveal their achievements and resources. That depth of engagement was necessary to inform future strategies for the organisation. Equally, it required the university researchers' knowledge of research methodologies to adapt the conceptual and analytical frameworks in response to the critical challenges from the participants. In the case of the CID, collaborative research was important to the purpose of the research because the project required researchers who were familiar with the content of the programme and the range of possible inclusive methods required to inform formative research processes. Again, an established history of collaboration benefited the effectiveness of the research, when shaping critical feedback from the findings and adjusting methods as the programme adapted to the findings.

The form of enquiry in both cases adopted inclusive methods in both research and evaluation. The university researchers included people with disabilities, as leaders, employees and advisors, in paid positions in the research teams. The organisations also allocated staff and members with disabilities to participate in the evaluation processes, including as advisors, researchers or participants. The impact of this inclusive approach was mutual and far-reaching, changing the research capacity of the community organisations and the capacity of the university researchers to use inclusive methods. The researchers and collaborators with lived experience filled the knowledge and practice gaps of the academic research team members.

The collaborative research approach adopted in each case endeavoured to utilise Cousin et al.'s three dimensions of collaborative inquiry (control of technical decision-making in the research; diversity in the range of stakeholders engaged; and depth of participation in the methodological elements of the research) through the inclusive membership of the research teams in the university and organisations, and through the inclusive methods, such as accessible design processes, data collection and forms of communication. These inclusive methods avoided reliance on written data collection by incorporating visual methods and discussions with peers. Outputs included easy-read materials with images and simple language. These methods were also adopted by the CID programme itself.

To be successful, research collaboration with Disabled Persons Organisations potentially must address all three of Cousins *et al.*'s research purposes (the practical, the political and the philosophical). The mission of Disabled Persons Organisations, particularly in the CRPD context, is one of addressing the practical needs of their members, the political representation of members' rights, and advocacy for a rights-based understanding of the experience of disability. These cases demonstrate that if researchers are personally familiar with the benefits of inclusive practice, they can incorporate these considerations into research design and conduct. In fact, they can intentionally adopt a research design process to shift power and decisions towards the Disabled Persons Organisations, thereby contributing to the achievement of important justice goals.

Beyond these two cases, we as authors have witnessed a broader change over the last two decades, as collaborative, inclusive research increasingly becomes expected by government and Disabled Persons Organisations in disability policy research. This change is partly a response to government obligations articulated in the CRPD, but it is also a result of the solidarity that has developed between Disabled Persons Organisations and researchers as advocates for the effectiveness of this approach. Disabled Persons Organisations have seen the benefit of using research for advocacy and lobbying, especially when the research uses a human rights or justice frame and adopts inclusive methods.

The success of research projects in influencing policy and practice change demonstrates that collaborative research is worth pursuing. It does, however, raise questions about feasibility. In an academic context, researchers are familiar with the additional pressures that this approach can introduce, exacerbating constraints on research from resource-sharing, time, academic performance and status, and any residual expectations from government officials more familiar with traditional 'independent' research. Disabled Persons Organisations recognise the time and resource pressures collaborative research requires. Research has not been traditionally seen as within their purview and current approaches to research and funding limit the ability of organisations to collaborate without increased resources and research capacity. For policymakers, collaborative research requires a broader perspective in terms of how research is initiated and funded and the outcome objectives identified.

These two case studies and our earlier research (Robinson *et al.* 2014) attest to the importance of reflective practice in the collaboration to address the tendency of these pressures to reproduce the injustices of exclusion of people with disabilities from research processes, particularly Cousin *et al.*'s third dimension of collaboration, which concerns the depth of participation in the methodological elements of the research. Time, and the budget consequences of needing more time, are the most obvious pressures in this regard. For example, in the second case study described here, the research team and the CID needed to discuss whether to delay data collection so that there was sufficient time to gather inclusive advice about aspects of the survey design.

More generally, academic researchers need to invest in the infrastructure to make collaborative, inclusive research possible. It is one thing for an individual researcher to develop a pattern of collaboration with a Disabled Persons Organisation or a person with disabilities. It is quite another for academics in general to attempt to shift research decision power towards the disability community, not least because of the historical exclusion of people with disabilities from tertiary education and research. Universities need to invest in mutual capacity of their researchers and Disabled Persons Organisations to develop new practices to work together. This will include developing relationships with Disabled Persons Organisations, enabling the tertiary education of people with disabilities, and employing people with disabilities more extensively in research and teaching.

Acknowledgements

We thank Shona Bates, Marie Delaney, Christine Eastman, Saul Flaxman, Andrew Griffiths, Ariella Meltzer, Peter Perry, Sally Robinson, Charlotte Smedley, Robert Strike, the NSW Council for Intellectual Disability, and Spinal Cord Injury Australia. Ethics approval for the research described in this chapter was provided by UNSW Sydney.

References

Australian Government, 2012. *Social Inclusion in Australia: How Australia is Faring.* 2nd edition. Canberra: Australian Social Inclusion Board.

Bates, S., Kayess, R. and Fisher, K. R., 2013. *Research into Maximising Life Choices of People with a Spinal Cord Injury, for Spinal Cord Injuries Australia.* SPRC Report 01/13. Sydney: Social Policy Research Centre, UNSW Sydney.

Charlton, J. I., 1998. *Nothing About Us Without Us: Disability Oppression and Empowerment.* Berkeley: University of California Press.

Committee on the Rights of Persons with Disabilities (CRPD), n.d. *Concluding Observations.* Geneva: United Nations. Available from: www.ohchr.org/EN/HRBodies/CRPD/Pages/CRPDIndex.aspx.

Cousins, J. B., Shulha, L. M., Whitmore, E., Al Hudib, H. andGlibert, N., 2016. How Do Evaluators Differentiate Successful from Less-than-Successful Experiences with Collaborative Approaches to Evaluation? *Evaluation Review*, 40 (1), 3–28.

Degener, T., 2016. Disability in a Human Rights Context. *Laws*, 5, 35.

Eurostat, 2014. *Eurostat Disability Statistics: Access to Education and Training.* Luxembourg: Eurostat. Available from: http://ec.europa.eu/eurostat/statistics-explained/index.php/Disability_statistics_-_access_to_education_and_training#Tertiary_education_completion:_those_with_disabilities_far_from_the_objective_of_40.C2.A0.25.

Fredman, S., 2011. *Discrimination Law.* 2nd edition. Oxford: Oxford University Press.

Griffiths, A., Nethery, D., Robinson, S., Bates, S., Kidd, E. and Kayess, R., 2017. *My Choice Matters Evaluation: Stage 4 and Final Report.* SPRC Report 05/17. Sydney: Social Policy Research Centre, UNSW Sydney.

Kayess, R., forthcoming. Equality and Inclusive Education. In: G. De Beco, S. Quinlivan and J. Lord, eds, *The Right to Inclusive Education in International Human Rights Law.* Cambridge: Cambridge University Press.

Kayess, R. and Smith, B., 2016. Human Rights Charters and Disability. In: C. Campbell, ed., *Australian Charters of Rights a Decade on.* Sydney: Federation Press, chapter 10.

Linton, S., 1998. *Claiming Disability: Knowledge and Identity.* New York: NYU Press.

Meltzer, A., Bates, S., Griffiths, A., Fisher, K., Kayess, R. and Robinson S., 2013. *My Choice Matters Evaluation Plan.* SPRC Report 9/13. Sydney: NSW Council for Intellectual Disability, Social Policy Research Centre, University of New South Wales.

Mertens, D., 2009. *Transformative Research and Evaluation.* New York: Guilford.

Nind, M. and Vinha, H., 2014. Doing Research Inclusively: Bridges to Multiple Possibilities in Inclusive Research. *British Journal of Learning Disability*, 42, 102–109.

OECD, 2011. *Inclusion of Students with Disabilities in Tertiary Education and Employment.* Paris: OECD Publishing. Available from: www.oecd.org/edu/innovation-education/inclusionofstudentswithdisabilitiesintertiaryeducationandemployment.htm

Ollerton, J. and Horsfall, D., 2013. Rights to Research: Utilising the Convention on the Rights of Persons with Disabilities as an Inclusive Participatory Action Research Tool. *Disability & Society*, 28 (5), 616–630.

Robinson, S., Fisher, K. R. and Strike, R., 2014. Participatory and Inclusive Approaches to Disability Policy Evaluation. *Australian Social Work*, 67 (4), 495–508.

Rogers, P. J. and Fraser, D., 2003. Appreciating Appreciative Inquiry. In: H. Preskill and A. T. Coghlan, eds, *Using Appreciative Inquiry in Evaluation.* San Francisco, CA: Jossey-Bass, 75–84.

Walmsley, J. and Johnson, K., 2003. *Inclusive Research with People with Learning Disabilities: Past, Present and Future.* London: Jessica Kingsley.

Weaver, L. and Cousins, J. B., 2004. Unpacking the Participatory Process. *Journal of Multidisciplinary Evaluation*, 1 (1), 19–40.

World Health Organization, 2011. *World Report on Disability: Chapter 7: Education.* Geneva: World Health Organization. Available from: www.who.int/disabilities/world_report/2011/report.pdf.

Chapter 11

Justice and the political future for Indigenous Australians

Darryl Cronin

Introduction

In the 1930s, the Aboriginal Australian activist William Cooper highlighted the importance of the Aboriginal voice and perspective in government policy because, in his view, white Australians could not 'think black' (Attwood and Markus 2004). Cooper and other Aboriginal activists were influential in developing an Indigenous political discourse around justice and rights, underpinned by the desire for freedom, justice and recognition of rights. Since the 1970s, this discourse has also encompassed notions of sovereignty and self-determination.

While the gains achieved to date have been piecemeal, recognition of rights, citizenship and land rights, for example, has enabled Indigenous people to make social, economic and political progress.[1] However, in the last two decades this progress has been undone or undermined by unsympathetic Australian governments. This undermining of the Indigenous rights approach has restrained Indigenous voices and Indigenous political power. Consequently, there exists no clear Indigenous political and philosophical road map for the future. In this regard, there is a need for political resurgence.

This chapter presents an Indigenous perspective of justice by discussing key issues in the context of recognition and reconciliation politics, drawing some conclusions about what the political future for Indigenous peoples in Australia might entail. The challenge for Indigenous Australians is to develop a resurgent political culture that challenges colonialism but which also balances social and economic development with obligations and responsibilities to country, community and cultural values.[2]

Justice and rights

Justice for Indigenous people includes claims for citizenship rights (the legal, political and social rights of citizens) and Indigenous rights (the culturally specific rights related to prior occupation). Indigenous rights are inherent to Indigenous cultural, spiritual and political traditions and include rights to self-determination, culture and land. There is a clear connection between justice and rights for Indigenous people because rectifying past injustice requires addressing current disadvantage and inequality, recognition of political status and recognising Indigenous customs, heritage and property rights. Justice, however, for Indigenous Australians has largely been limited to addressing Indigenous inequality and socio-economic disadvantage through distributive measures. The broader issue of addressing historical wrongs of colonisation through restorative, reparative or relational forms of justice has largely been rejected by successive Australian governments. Unlike other countries colonised by Britain, there were no treaties with Indigenous peoples in Australia.

The inability of Australian governments to address historical injustice or negotiate a different relationship with Indigenous people has its genesis in colonial assumptions and beliefs that deemed Indigenous people to have 'deficiencies' in respect to European society. Colonial discourse and practices regarded Indigenous Australians as having no organised societies, no land ownership or a recognisable form of sovereignty – the belief was that Indigenous people had to be 'civilised' through the erasure of their culture and their absorption into European ways of life. These incorrect assumptions spawned an array of negative and demeaning attitudes and beliefs about Indigenous people which remain ingrained in governmental institutions, Indigenous policymaking and contemporary public attitudes.

In his Lingiari Memorial Lecture in August 1999, Patrick Dodson (2000) outlined what he thought would provide justice for Indigenous people. This included rights to equality, freedom and distinct Indigenous rights; maintenance of Indigenous identities; political self-determination; recognition of Indigenous laws, customs and traditions; rights to religious and spiritual traditions; rights to language, stories, histories and traditions; measures to improve economic and social conditions; control of land, waters and resources; self-government and autonomy; constitutional recognition; and a legislative framework for agreements and negotiation (Dodson 2000, pp. 65–76). Similar measures had been proposed in the earlier 1988 *Barunga Statement* and the 1993 *Eva Valley Statement*. Both statements emphasised the protection of Indigenous rights, culture and heritage within a human rights framework and control of decision-making through consultation, negotiation and consent (Behrendt 2003, pp. 86–90).

The *Aboriginal Peace Plan* presented to Prime Minister Paul Keating in April 1993 called for a long-term settlement with Indigenous people including constitutional recognition. The 2017 *Uluru Statement from the Heart* emphasised Indigenous ownership of land, the basis of sovereignty that has never been ceded and which continues to co-exist with the sovereignty of the Crown. The statement called for the establishment of a First Nation voice enshrined in the Australian Constitution and a Makarrata Commission to supervise agreement-making between Australian governments and First Nations and oversee historical truth-telling (Commonwealth of Australia 2017).[3]

Indigenous struggles

During the protection and assimilation era that characterised early relations between the colonisers and Indigenous peoples, struggles centred on recognising Indigenous identity and culture, gaining citizenship rights and land rights. In colonial Victoria in the late 1800s, Aboriginal people were considered inferior and a doomed race; however, the people living on Coranderrk reserve in the state of Victoria challenged oppressive policies of 'protection' and agitated for equality, freedom and rights to lands. In the 1930s–1940s, Aboriginal people were considered not 'civilised' enough to be citizens or capable of making progress towards 'civilisation'. However, in 1938 Aboriginal activists in Sydney used the Australian celebration of the 150th anniversary of the landing of the First Fleet to stage a day of mourning conference to appeal to the conscience of Australians about the plight of Aboriginal people and to agitate for citizenship and land rights. In 1963, the Yolngu people in Arnhem Land were considered inferior and unintelligent, but they drew on their cultural values to challenge the imposition of a bauxite mine on their traditional country and to assert their ownership of land and protection of culture. In 1972, Indigenous activists in Redfern, Sydney drew inspiration from the Black Power movement in the USA to establish an Aboriginal Embassy in Canberra, defying parliamentary authority and embarrassing the federal government, calling for land rights, self-determination and a treaty. Their protest paved the way for the Australian Government to implement a policy of self-determination that allowed Indigenous communities to make their own decisions about their social and economic futures. This self-determination policy enabled Indigenous leaders in the 1980s to call for national land rights and a treaty with Indigenous people as well as seek a greater political voice into government policymaking. These Indigenous claims became public policy initiatives, but the Australian Government abandoned them. Instead, in the 1990s it instituted a formal process of reconciliation whereby the Australian nation would come to terms with its history and provide some redress to Indigenous people. But this reconciliation process failed to achieve better outcomes for Indigenous people, having marginalised treaty and sovereignty together with other issues important to Indigenous people (Gunstone 2007, pp. 146–158, 302–303).

The recognition of native title rights to land in 1992 by the Australian High Court in its *Mabo* judgment[4] and subsequent Indigenous negotiations with the federal government regarding native title legislation enabled Indigenous people to regain some of their traditional country. However, the 1993 negotiations with the federal government were conducted in a public political environment that considered Indigenous people and their rights inferior. The Australian Government took an extinguishment approach whereby it developed legislation to validate non-Indigenous land titles and to restrict native title. Such a stance was consolidated in 1996 when the Australian Government under Prime Minister John Howard abandoned the policy of self-determination, dismantled national Indigenous representation, undermined Indigenous authority and political voices, and introduced an individual responsibility paradigm into policy and practice (MacDonald and Muldoon 2006, pp. 216–220). Among other things, the Howard Government dismantled the Aboriginal and Torres Strait Islander Commission, amended the *Native Title Act* 1993 to restrict the rights of native title holders, launched a military intervention into Northern Territory Aboriginal communities, refused to apologise to the stolen generations, voted against the UN Declaration on the Rights of Indigenous Peoples, and derailed the formal reconciliation process. These events systematically undermined Indigenous political voice and resulted in the rejection of Indigenous political authority and agency.

Discrediting Indigenous self-determination

The impact of the upheaval of Indigenous affairs in 1996 still reverberates today. The Howard Government promoted the narrative that Indigenous self-determination had failed, therefore coercive intervention was required (Dodson 2007, p. 23). Indigenous voices also questioned the Indigenous rights approach because of the continuing impoverishment of Indigenous communities and the levels of violence, particularly against women and children. Noel Pearson, for example, a prominent Indigenous leader, questioned why there has been significant social and cultural deterioration in Indigenous communities during a period of Indigenous policy enlightenment and recognition (Pearson 2009, p. 173). Pearson claimed that social breakdown and cultural fragmentation in communities is created by Indigenous dependence on welfare income from government, which creates a passive welfare economy devoid of any reciprocation or responsibility, and this in turn entrenches abusive and destructive behaviour (Pearson 2009, pp. 146–153, 234).

But other Indigenous leaders and intellectuals disputed that all Indigenous communities are dysfunctional. Dysfunction and social breakdown may have become more noticeable, but it has been around since British-Australian colonisation and was entrenched by policies of protection and assimilation as well as attitudes of racism and beliefs in

Indigenous inferiority. History shows, however, that Indigenous agency and struggle have been central to resisting the exterminatory and assimilatory policies and practices of government. Since the 1970s, Indigenous struggles for justice have encompassed notions of sovereignty and self-determination in line with the principles enshrined in Article 3 of the United Nations Declaration on the Rights of Indigenous Peoples, which specifically states that self-determination is a right of Indigenous people to freely determine their political status and pursue their economic, social and cultural development.

Indigenous sovereignty

Sovereignty, according to Michael Mansell, 'goes to the heart of the Aboriginal struggle', sustaining land rights, customary law and self-determination, and is expressed through traditional authority (Mansell 2016, p. 74). In contrast, Marcia Langton has argued that Indigenous people have not clearly articulated how sovereignty might be achieved, hence it remains a slogan (Langton 2012, pp. 138–139). While there is need for clarity, Mansell says that Aboriginal calls for sovereignty are a reminder that the source of Indigenous entitlement derives from Aboriginal sovereignty, not government policy (Mansell 2016, pp. 183–184).

In that regard the Indigenous use of the word 'sovereignty' is deliberate to 'convey a sense of prior and fundamental authority' as well as signify the inherent power of Indigenous people to determine their futures which is not granted by the Australian Constitution or any settler document or institution (Brennan *et al.* 2004, p. 316). Larissa Behrendt has supported this notion, stating Indigenous sovereignty claims demand rights and the devolution of power from the Australian state; they are not about threatening its sovereignty (Behrendt 2003, pp. 99, 115). Phillip Falk and Gary Martin agree that Indigenous sovereignty is an assertion of internal sovereignty comparable with the 'domestic dependent nation' status of Indigenous people in North America. They contend that the conclusion of a treaty or treaties with the Australian Government is an essential hallmark in this respect (Falk and Martin 2007, pp. 39, 45). Calls for a treaty, however, are not new. The issue of treaty was formally taken up by the National Aboriginal Conference in 1979, who argued that Aboriginal people should be recognised as a 'domestic dependent nation'. They adopted the term Makarrata and undertook Australia-wide consultations with Indigenous people. But the Australian Government at the time was never committed to a treaty. Treaty was again placed on the public policy agenda in June 1988 when Prime Minister Bob Hawke promised a treaty, but in the face of conservative opposition Hawke retreated and instead proposed reconciliation.

Recognition and reconciliation politics

Since the 1970s, successive Australian governments have attempted to accommodate Indigenous claims by way of a politics of recognition – a political approach used by settler states to accommodate and reconcile Indigenous identity claims and Indigenous assertions of nationhood with settler state sovereignty (Coulthard 2014, p. 151). The recognition of land rights and native title offer examples of this. The formal recognition of Indigenous people in the Australian Constitution is a contemporary public policy issue. In November 2010 the Australian Government established an expert panel to determine the best option for an amendment to the Australian Constitution to recognise Aboriginal and Torres Strait Islander peoples. It recommended the repeal of potentially discriminatory provisions of the Constitution (section 25 and 51 (xxxvi)) and the insertion of new sections (section 51A and 116A) to enable the parliament to make laws for Indigenous people and to prohibit discrimination based on race (Commonwealth of Australia 2012, pp. 153, 173).

In March 2013, the Australian parliament passed the *Aboriginal and Torres Strait Islander Peoples Recognition Act 2013* to symbolically recognise Indigenous people as the first inhabitants of the Australian continent; it also provided for a review of progress on constitutional recognition. A Parliamentary Joint Select Committee on Constitutional Recognition of Aboriginal and Torres Strait Islander Peoples was established soon after. In June 2015, the joint select committee recommended that a referendum be held to recognise Indigenous people in the Constitution. It also recommended repeal and recasting of potentially discriminatory provisions in the Constitution (section 25 and section 51xxvi) and set out three options to progress to a successful referendum (Commonwealth of Australia 2015).

At the same time the government established and funded 'Recognise', a public relations campaign to lobby for a 'Yes' vote in a referendum even though there was no referendum proposal. This raised the suspicions of Indigenous people. According to Celeste Little, 'Recognise' was no more than an ad campaign to 'peddle the government's agenda' (Liddle 2014). Ghillar Michael Anderson, who opposed the referendum, said it was 'criminally deceitful' for the Recognise campaign to ask people to support a referendum to change the Constitution without a final form of words for a referendum question (Anderson 2014). By 2014 the focus and process of constitutional recognition began to stagnate, and the review panel established under the Recognition Act 2013 noted this. Indigenous people were becoming frustrated by the delays and perceived lack of government commitment for constitutional recognition. There was a loss of public momentum and awareness of the issue of constitutional recognition and so the review panel said Australians were not ready for a referendum. It recommended a Referendum Council to finalise a proposal for constitutional amendment and that a referendum be held no later than the first half of 2017 (Anderson *et al.* 2014). According to Megan Davis and Marcia Langton, the drift in the constitutional recognition debate, the lack of a model for constitutional recognition and the promotion of a 'softer version of reform' by the Recognise campaign inspired Indigenous resistance (Davis and Langton 2016, p. 5).

Throughout, the Australian Government had been managing the process to achieve an outcome based on what would be acceptable to them and its conservative constituency. This became clear in July 2015 when then Prime Minister Tony Abbott and Opposition Leader Bill Shorten hosted 40 handpicked Indigenous leaders to discuss a way forward. Indigenous leaders requested an Indigenous process to enable an Indigenous consensus on a model for recognition, but this was rejected by the prime minister, only for him to change his mind some weeks later following meetings with Indigenous leaders. Noel Pearson said the process for going forward had been predetermined by the government because two ideas not discussed in the meeting were the key outcome: that of broad community conferences with no mention of the need for Indigenous conferences; and a Referendum Council, which most Indigenous leaders had not heard of (Pearson 2015). The Australian Government wants only minimal constitutional change. Issues such as recognition of Indigenous sovereignty, self-determination and treaty are deemed not acceptable for consideration in a referendum proposal since they are issues that Australians refuse to address. The expert panel made this clear in 2012 when it said the issue of Indigenous sovereignty would be 'highly contested' and any constitutional backing for a treaty would likely confuse Australians and therefore likely jeopardise public support for the panel's recommendations (Commonwealth of Australia 2012, pp. 201, 213).

As issues of Indigenous sovereignty and treaty were not addressed, 'recognition' in the Constitution has become meaningless for many Indigenous people. Mansell has argued that Aboriginal people never needed to be recognised to establish prior occupation, so why is there a need for recognition by white Australians? He maintains that Indigenous recognition will not alter the institutional arrangements established by the Australian Constitution (Davis and Langton 2016, pp. 145–154). Nayuka Gorrie points out that recognition is something bestowed upon Indigenous people by white Australians to legitimise their colonial system, whereas 'treaties are legal mechanisms between two parties that recognise one another's sovereignty' (Gorrie 2016). Gorrie's point is important because it explains why there is so strong an Indigenous resistance to constitutional recognition.

The constitutional recognition agenda is more about reforming the Australian Constitution. However, aspirations of constitutional reform were overtaken by so-called 'constitutional conservatives' who vowed to oppose any proposal that entrench rights in the Constitution (Craven 2016, p. 38). Noel Pearson has attempted to find a middle ground between such a position and Indigenous aspirations for constitutional change. He proposed an alternative constitutional amendment to enable Indigenous people to have a say about laws and policies made about them. Parliament would create the Indigenous representative mechanism and symbolic statements of recognition would be achieved through a declaration outside of the Constitution (Davis and Langton 2016, p. 174). But Michael Mansell says Pearson's proposal risks the 'constitutional entrenchment of subordination' and it cannot be described as a step towards self-determination (Mansell 2016, p. 53).

The limits of recognition

The constitutional recognition of Indigenous Australians can only be granted by a majority of Australians in a majority of states who vote in a referendum. As a minority, Aboriginal and Torres Strait Islander peoples have no voting power nor real influence over the democratic processes. Politicians determine the political processes and a majority of the population will decide whether they want to recognise Indigenous peoples. Nevertheless, Indigenous people have been able to formulate and present their proposal regarding constitutional change to the government because of a national engagement and consultation programme conducted with Indigenous peoples between December 2016 and May 2017 by a Referendum Council.

The Referendum Council was established to advise on the steps to a successful referendum. During these dialogues, the proposal for an Indigenous voice in the Constitution along with the constitutional reforms proposed by the expert panel were discussed. In its recommendations of June 2017, the Referendum Council said a referendum should be held to provide for an Indigenous representative voice to the Australian parliament in the Australian Constitution and that all Australian parliaments enact legislation to articulate a symbolic statement of recognition. Importantly, although the issue of treaty was not part of the original expert panel reforms, proposals for a treaty or agreement-making mechanism were strongly endorsed by the Indigenous dialogues (Commonwealth of Australia 2017, pp. 2, 14). The Indigenous dialogues advanced a different view from that of the expert panel. Indigenous people were not persuaded by the benefits of a statement of acknowledgement in the Constitution, nor were they supportive of removing potentially discriminatory clauses from the Constitution as they would confer no substantive benefit and the issues were considered low priority in many dialogues or rejected by other dialogues. There was ambivalence regarding a prohibition against adverse discrimination; however, the dialogues supported a constitutionally entrenched voice to parliament and an agreement-making mechanism such as a treaty. The need for truth-telling about Australia's history of colonisation was also stressed. An Indigenous voice enshrined in the Constitution and a Makarrata Commission to supervise truth-telling and agreement-making between governments and Indigenous people were proposals later endorsed by a National Indigenous Constitutional Convention at Uluru in May 2017 (Commonwealth of Australia 2017, pp. 10–28).

When the Australian Government considered the recommendations of the Referendum Council in October 2017, it rejected the idea of a national Indigenous representative voice to parliament. Prime Minister Malcolm Turnbull said it was a 'radical change' to the Constitution and was not 'desirable or capable of winning acceptance in a referendum'. He also said the proposal was inconsistent with a fundamental principle of Australian democracy: namely, that Australian citizens have equal civic rights to vote for, stand for and serve in the national parliament (Turnbull 2017). Indigenous representatives were enraged that the government had once again let Indigenous people down and that the prime minister could be so disrespectful by dictating what form Indigenous recognition should take. The government believed the Indigenous representative assembly proposal stood little chance of success yet offered no evidence in that regard. Their opposition to the proposal was more ideological, being driven by colonial views about the place of Indigenous people in the Australian nation. This was reflected in their opinion that an Indigenous body would be a third chamber of parliament and inconsistent with Australian democratic principle.

There can be no democracy for Indigenous people in Australia so long as Indigenous people are consistently on the losing side of majority decision-making processes. Constitutional democracy was established to serve the rights and interests of the majority population. As a minority, Indigenous people do not have equal access to or influence over government policy and decision-making. Based on what Indigenous people have experienced and seen over the course of history, the 'politics of recognition' has achieved very little or has only achieved piecemeal outcomes for Indigenous people. Constitutional recognition is going down a similar path to that of the formal reconciliation process (1991–2000), which failed because political reconciliation with Indigenous people was not considered necessary by the Australian Government.

The Canadian Aboriginal scholar Glen Coulthard argues that 'recognition' does not significantly modify the power in colonial relationships because ultimately it is conceived as something that is 'granted' to a subordinate group by a dominant group (Coulthard 2014, pp. 30–31). Coulthard's criticism echoes the criticisms of Indigenous people in Australia towards constitutional recognition, but it also explains why the outcomes of incremental recognition of Indigenous claims throughout history have not transformed the colonial relationship between Indigenous people and successive Australian governments. Recognition politics has also been detrimental to the Indigenous struggle because it has encouraged Indigenous people to adopt conciliatory approaches on the basis that the government will reciprocate with goodwill. But politicians and governments are resistant to defending or promoting Indigenous rights. In that regard, constitutional recognition may not be the appropriate pathway at this time. Indigenous peoples may need to rethink the way forward.

Recognition and political power

A fundamental question for Aboriginal and Torres Strait Islander peoples is how best to achieve aspirations and objectives for justice within the political and constitutional framework of the colonial state. The proposal for an Indigenous representative voice to parliament and the negotiation of a treaty with Indigenous people are proposals put forward for Indigenous political participation in Australian government. However, the Australian Government says that a constitutionally entrenched Indigenous voice is a special privilege only for Indigenous people. But Indigenous people are asking for recognition of their sovereign status as first peoples as one way of acknowledging historical wrongs. The government believes Indigenous people should get elected to the Australian parliament to have a stronger voice. However, since the first sitting of the Australian parliament in 1901, there have only been ten Indigenous parliamentarians, seven of whom were elected to the Senate. Most of those Indigenous parliamentarians were elected after the year 2010.

Recognition of Indigenous political power within Australian government is largely confined to a minority of Indigenous politicians who represent mainstream political parties and government-appointed Indigenous advisory bodies. The Indigenous representative voice proposal endorsed by the Referendum Council is different because it will be constitutionally entrenched; therefore it cannot be abolished by government. Past and current Indigenous advisory bodies to government are often ineffective because they lack status, political power and influence and can be easily abolished by government. This is because mainstream politicians, public sector bureaucrats and other public decision-makers who represent the interests of the majority population determine what justice is for Indigenous peoples. Indigenous people therefore remain reliant on the goodwill of the majority and the power of mainstream politicians to grant recognition.

The Australian Government will not tolerate an Indigenous political authority in Australian constitutional government. For Indigenous people, political authority relates to the right to self-determination and this requires not only a structural shift but also a shift in the Australian mindset. Mick Dodson has said there must be a fundamental shift in the structure of power and this would involve building an Indigenous voice into Australian government and reforming the structural basis of excluding Indigenous people from state power (Dodson 1994, pp. 68, 72). Larissa Behrendt echoes such a perspective in arguing for institutional and structural reform of government to remove the power imbalance and to counter entrenched institutional ideologies and biases (Behrendt 2003, pp. 122–131). The structural reform of government, according to Megan Davis, requires a redistribution of public power of the state to make proper room for Indigenous peoples (Davis and Langton 2016, p. 88). Mansell argues that designated Indigenous seats in the Australian parliament would enhance democracy and he suggests 12 Indigenous seats in the Senate, the upper house of the Australian parliament (Mansell 2016, pp. 34–35). To heal the wounds of the past and contribute towards national unity and reconciliation, Mansell recommends a truth, justice and reconciliation commission (Mansell 2016, pp. 133–145). As a long-term vision, he also proposes a seventh Australian state that could be legislated for by the Australian Government and take the form of a treaty (Mansell 2016, pp. 198–224).

Given the minority status of Indigenous peoples and the lack of representation or influence in government, obtaining political power will involve seeking the support of a majority of the Australian population, many of whom have little understanding or awareness of colonisation and its impact on Indigenous people. It also includes gaining the support of political parties in the parliament, where Indigenous policy is subject to the political machinations of mainstream politics. Politicians hold allegiance to liberal government, whose traditions and conventions reinforce the constitutional systems and frameworks that have historically excluded Indigenous people and demeaned their cultural or political rights. A structural and psychological shift within Australian government and society may be a leap beyond the thinking and imagination of many Australians.

To challenge and overcome these historical and ideological barriers, Indigenous Australians need to rebuild an Indigenous political discourse around justice and rights. One practical way of doing this has been described as Indigenous resurgence, which in Canada has contributed to the growth of Indigenous political cultures. This resurgence, asserts Leanne Betasmosake Simpson, requires Indigenous people to grow up strongly connected to their land, immersed in their languages and spiritualities, and embodying their traditions of agency, leadership, decision-making and diplomacy (Simpson 2014). Taiaiake Alfred advocates for Indigenous Canadians to embrace traditional values to create legitimate forms of governance to drive the political relationship with the settler state. He argues that the removal of Indigenous people from land and the associated cultural disconnection and erosion of cultural values has created not only an economic and political dependency on the Canadian state, but also a psychological and spiritual dependency on the government's assimilative notion of what it means to be 'Canadian'. Therefore, Indigenous resurgence is founded in the need for Indigenous Canadians to re-establish themselves as cultural beings connected psychologically and spiritually to the land (Alfred 2015, pp. 5–8). Indigenous people need to break the bonds of dependency to create stability, autonomy and self-sufficiency and a culture that will insulate them from the continuing impacts of colonisation.

Also in Canada, Glen Coulthard argues that Indigenous societies can curb the assimilative and hegemonic power of the Canadian state by redirecting their struggle away from conciliatory forms of recognition politics towards a 'resurgent politics of recognition' premised upon Indigenous forms of self-recognition, direct action and the resurgence of cultural practices that pay close attention to settler-colonial power (Coulthard 2014, p. 24). This may be achieved through political-economic alternatives tied to the relationship in land; building solidarity between urban Aboriginal people and reserve-based First Nations for mutual empowerment; recognising the centrality of Aboriginal women and taking responsibility to end the violence against women; and engaging with the settler-state through critical self-reflection but also through direct action (Coulthard 2014, pp. 165–179).

Indigenous resurgence in Australia

Echoing many of the issues discussed above, Irene Watson argues that Indigenous Australians can only re-emerge with an assured future by restoring Indigenous humanity through the recognition of Indigenous philosophy and knowledge. This requires rethinking and articulating political possibilities beyond the existing frame of assimilation, unpacking claims concerning *terra nullius* through an Indigenous standpoint, and developing counter-narratives to neo-liberalism (Watson 2014, pp. 513, 517–519).[5] The dominant narrative in government Indigenous policy and Indigenous discourse over the last two decades has focused on individual responsibility, economic integration and tackling welfare dependency.

In contrast, Patrick Dodson argues for the reconstruction of Indigenous society through traditionally based governance structures, customary land ownership and internal reconciliation and healing to build social cohesion through the interconnected obligations and responsibilities (Dodson 2007, p. 24). Cultural structures and cultural values have always been important to the Yolngu people of north-east Arnhem Land, whose land and traditional existence have been impacted upon severely through bauxite mining. Their desire for a better future and the need to reconcile with the world is grounded deep in Yolngu culture. Galarrwuy Yunupingu explains that cultural obligations and responsibilities through song cycles, the ceremonies, the knowledge, the law and the land guide the life and essence of the Yolngu clans, keeping balance and giving meaning to people (Yunupingu 2008–09). Similarly, the Yawuru people in the town of Broome in Western Australia see the recognition of their native title rights as part of a journey to reconstruct their community after more than a century of colonisation and domination. They anchor their history and contemporary life in the country, the people, the language, the stories and the law that arises from country. These shape contemporary cultural prac-tices and values, relationships with country, and obligations and respons-ibilities. Central to Yawuru restoration is *mabu liyan (good spirit)* – in the form of the continuity and connection between the mind, body, spirit, culture and land (Yap and Yu 2016, p. 14). *Liyan* is expressed through emotional strength, dignity and pride.

Most especially, however, the restoration of Indigenous society must heed the knowledge, experience and voice of Indigenous women (Moreton-Robinson 2013). Suzanne Ingram contends that the voice of Aboriginal women regarding inequality and high rates of domestic viol-ence, for example, has been silenced by the privileging of other issues, and so the voice of Aboriginal women has been subsumed by the solidarity ideology of the Aboriginal movement (Ingram 2016, pp. 10–11).

Restoration and nationhood

Instilling Indigenous responsibility, reducing welfare dependency, and ameliorating economic problems all have a role to play in restoring Indigenous communities. However, Indigenous forms of restoration and development are not confined to these factors. Maintaining author-ity and cultural integrity are also vital as reflected in the actions of the Ngarrindjeri people in south-eastern South Australia, who have under-taken a nation-building programme. To respond to water planning issues on their traditional country, and using their native title rights in land, the Ngarrindjeri consolidated their governing authority into a regional authority based on traditional governance as the central point of administration and involvement in the government policy and plan-ning regimes. They also negotiated agreements with the state govern-ment that required listening, discussion and negotiation over all management matters concerning Ngarrindjeri people and their country. In support of these actions, the Ngarrindjeri developed a statement of principle which stresses the interconnectedness between health of country and health of people and cultural life. These principles shape policy and practice and enable the Ngarrindjeri to speak with cultural specificity and authority as to their country, serving as the basis for respectful and positive intercultural partnerships that recognise Indigenous rights (Rigney *et al.* 2015, pp. 334–349).

The Ngarrindjeri, the Yawuru, the Yolngu and other Indigenous groups are grounding their development and restoration in their traditional ways of knowing, being and doing. Their actions align with the Indigenous development paradigm whereby Indigenous people gain political authority by reorganising themselves as peoples in accordance with their ideals. Nation-building assists Indigenous groups to reclaim their traditional country or reconstruct their traditional boundaries, rebuild their collective identity, traditions, culture and political organisations and assert self-governing authority. An essential step of nation-building is to act as a nation and create governance organisations to make and implement decisions on behalf of the group, resolve disputes, build and sustain productive intergovernmental relationships with outside entities as well as accept responsibility for delivering goods and revitalising culture (Cornell 2015). For Indigenous Australians, nation-building can strengthen authority, as well as identity and culture. It can reinforce the importance of obligations and responsibilities within communities and enable a political voice that is anchored in Indigenous values and ideals.

The challenge ahead

The Indigenous future in Australia involves a continuation of historical struggles for justice and rights. It must include protest and conflict. Without conflict and struggle, the terms of recognition tend to remain with those in possession of power to bestow in ways they deem appropriate (Coulthard 2014, p. 39) However, since the 1990s it has become apparent that a rethink is required on how best to renew Indigenous Australian political discourse and strategy because there is no one Indigenous political approach or political philosophy that has the broad support of Indigenous people. Aboriginal and Torres Strait Islander peoples know what they want; however, there is not enough intellectual focus on how these aspirations might be achieved given their minority status in a colonial state.

Indigenous leaders and intellectuals play a critical role in renewing political discourse and strategy. In doing so, they must not only defend Indigenous rights and authority but must also engage and challenge the legal and political discourses of government and society that constrain or resist Indigenous self-determination. This requires resisting contemporary forms of colonialism; confronting the hegemony and inertia of Australian legal, political and economic institutions; asserting a stake in political and public discussions about Indigenous policy; defending and protecting the integrity of Indigenous rights and Indigenous ways of knowing; and finding alternative ways of engaging with mainstream Australian society and government over questions of justice and rights. Importantly, Indigenous leaders and intellectuals must promote Indigenous values and ideals, and this requires rebuilding or strengthening Indigenous authority and cultural integrity within communities.

The challenge for the future therefore lies in articulating a political and philosophical roadmap which not only promotes an Indigenous future, but which sets out how this future should be achieved. Colonialism exists and needs to be challenged, being embodied in political and philosophical frameworks of government in Australia. An Indigenous political resurgence involves reclaiming political and cultural authority and finding innovative ways of challenging or changing Australian political culture to assert rights, pursue justice and find solutions to community problems and issues. This requires challenging government recognition and reconciliation approaches and developing alternative approaches that give power to Indigenous people rather than accepting strategies that are more about cleansing the conscience of Australians.

Notes

1 While it is preferable to use the term 'Aboriginal and Torres Strait Islander Peoples' to describe the Indigenous peoples of Australia, I use the term 'Indigenous' interchangeably with the term 'Aboriginal' throughout.
2 For Indigenous Australians, the English word 'country' denotes a cultural and spiritual place to which they have strong connections. Indigenous Australians speak of their traditional country which can refer to land or sea/water. 'Country' is a political and cultural entity that defines and determines law, culture, identity, kinship, relationships and obligations.
3 *Makarrata* is a Yolngu word from north-east Arnhem Land which is described as meaning 'a coming together after a struggle', to settle a dispute.
4 *Mabo and Others v The State of Queensland* [No. 2] [1992] 175 Commonwealth Law Report, 1.
5 *Terra nullius* literally means land belonging to no one. Its use justified the British acquisition of sovereignty over the Australian continent, thus dispossessing Indigenous peoples. *Terra nullius* lands were regarded as either wholly unoccupied or occupied by people who were considered to have no legal, social and political system worthy of recognition.

References

Alfred, T., 2015. Cultural Strength: Restoring the Place of Indigenous Knowledge in Practice and Policy. *Australian Aboriginal Studies*, 1, 3–11.
Anderson, G. M., 2014. *The Government is Asking You to Blindly Vote for Changes in a Referendum, without Even Clarifying the Final Wording*. Available from: http://nationalunitygovernment.org/content/government-asking-you-blindly-vote-changes-referendum-without-even-clarifying-final-wording [Accessed 26 April 2018].

Anderson, J., Hosch, T. and Eccles. R., 2014. *Final Report of the Aboriginal and Torres Strait Islander Act of Recognition Review Panel*, September 2014. Canberra, ACT: Department of Prime Minister and Cabinet, Australian Government.

Attwood, B. and Markus, A., 2004. *Thinking Black: William Cooper and the Australian Aborigines' League*. Canberra, ACT: Aboriginal Studies Press.

Behrendt, L., 2003. *Achieving Social Justice: Indigenous Rights and Australia's Future*. Annandale, NSW: The Federation Press.

Brennan, S., Gunn, B. and Williams, G., 2004. Sovereignty and Its Relevance to Treaty-Making between Indigenous Peoples and Australian Governments. *Sydney Law Review*, 26, 307–352.

Commonwealth of Australia, 2012. *Recognising Aboriginal and Torres Strait Islander Peoples in the Constitution: Report of the Expert Panel*, January 2012. Canberra, ACT: Department of Families, Housing, Community Services and Indigenous Affairs.

Commonwealth of Australia, 2015. *Joint Select Committee on Constitutional Recognition of Aboriginal and Torres Strait Islander Peoples: Final Report*, June 2015. Canberra, ACT: Parliament House.

Commonwealth of Australia, 2017. *Final Report of the Referendum Council*, 30 June 2017. Canberra, ACT: Department of Prime Minister and Cabinet.

Cornell, S., 2015. Processes of Native Nationhood: The Indigenous Politics of Self-Government. *The International Indigenous Policy Journal*, 6 (4), Article 4, 1–26.

Coulthard, G. S., 2014. *Red Skin White Masks: Rejecting the Colonial Politics of Recognition*. Minneapolis, MN: University of Minnesota Press.

Craven, G., 2016. The Law, Substance and Morality of Recognition. In: D. Freeman and S. Morris, eds, *The Forgotten People: Liberal and Conservative Approaches to Recognising Indigenous Peoples*. Carlton, VIC: Melbourne University Press, 31–40.

Davis, M. and Langton, M., eds, 2016. *It's Our Country: Indigenous Arguments for Meaningful Constitutional Recognition and Reform*. Carlton, VIC: Melbourne University Press.

Dodson, M., 1994. Towards the Exercise of Indigenous Rights: Policy, Power and Self-determination, *Race & Class*, 35 (4), 65–76.

Dodson, P., 2000. Until the Chains are Broken, 1999 Vincent Lingiari Memorial Lecture. *Australian Indigenous Law Reporter*, 5 (2), 73–84.

Dodson, P., 2007. Whatever Happened to Reconciliation. In: J. Altman and M. Hinkson, eds, *Coercive Reconciliation: Stabilise, Normalise, Exit Aboriginal Australia*. North Carlton, VIC: Arena Publications, 21–29.

Falk, P. and Martin, G., 2007. Misconstruing Indigenous Sovereignty: Maintaining the Fabric of Australian Law. In: A. Moreton-Robinson, ed., *Sovereign Subjects, Indigenous Sovereignty Matters*. Crows Nest, NSW: Allen & Unwin, 33–46.

Gorrie, N., 2016. *Fuck Your Constitutional Recognition, I Want a Treaty*. VICE [online]. Available from: www.vice.com/en_au/article/qb5zdp/fuck-your-recognition [Accessed 26 April 2018].

Gunstone, A., 2007. *Unfinished Business: The Australian Formal Reconciliation Process*. Melbourne, VIC: Australian Scholarly Publishing.

Ingram, S., 2016. Silent Drivers: Driving Silence – Aboriginal Women's Voices on Domestic Violence. *Social Alternatives*, 35 (1), 6–12.

Langton, M., 2012. *The Quiet Revolution: Indigenous People and the Resources Boom*. Boyer Lectures 2012. Sydney, NSW: ABC Books.

Liddle, C., 2014. I Don't Want Your Recognise Campaign – It's Nothing but a Sham. *Guardian*, 18 August. Available from: www.theguardian.com/commentisfree/2014/

aug/18/i-dont-want-your-recognise-campaign-its-nothing-but-a-sham [Accessed 26 April 2018].

MacDonald, L. T. O. T. and Muldoon, P., 2006. Globalisation, Neo-liberalism and the Struggle for Indigenous Citizenship. *Australian Journal of Political Science*, 41 (2), 209–233.

Mansell, M., 2016. *Treaty and Statehood: Aboriginal Self-Determination*. Leichhardt, NSW: The Federation Press.

Moreton-Robinson, A., 2013. Towards an Australian Indigenous Women's Standpoint Theory. *Australian Feminist Studies*, 28 (78), 331–347.

Pearson, N., 2009. *Up from the Mission*. Melbourne, VIC: Black Inc.

Pearson, N., 2015. Process of Recognition: The Constitutional Recognition of Indigenous Australians Requires Meaningful Consultation. *The Monthly*, August 2015. Available from: www.themonthly.com.au/issue/2015/august/1438351200/noel-pearson/process-recognition [Accessed 26 April 2018].

Rigney, D., Bignall, S. and Hemming, S., 2015. Negotiating Indigenous Modernity: Kungun Ngarrindjeri Yunnan – Listen to Ngarrindjeri Speak. *AlterNative: An International Journal of Indigenous Peoples*, 11 (4), 334–349.

Simpson, L. B., 2014. Land as Pedagogy: Nishnaabeg Intelligence and Rebellious Transformation. *Decolonization: Indigeneity, Education & Society*, 3 (3), 1–25.

Turnbull, M., 2017. *Response to Referendum Council's Report on Constitutional Recognition*. Media Release Malcolm Turnbull MP, 26 October.

Watson, I., 2014. Re-centring First Nations Knowledge and Places in a Terra Nullius Space. *AlterNative: An International Journal of Indigenous Peoples*, 10 (5) 508–520.

Yap, M. and Yu, E., 2016. Foreword by Patrick Dodson, *Community Wellbeing from the Ground up: A Yawuru Example*, Report No. 3/16 August. Bently, WA: Bankwest Curtin Economics Centre.

Yunupingu, G., 2008–09. Tradition, Truth & Tomorrow. *The Monthly*, December 2008–January 2009, 32–40.

Chapter 12

The serendipity of justice

The case of unaccompanied migrant children becoming 'adult' in the UK

Elaine Chase

Introduction

Prior to 2015, an average of around 12,000 migrant children without any accompanying adult arrived in Europe each year. The refugee crisis in 2015 witnessed an unprecedented 90,000 such children arriving during a 12-month period. The UK receives several thousand such children each year who, on arrival, are systematically channelled through the asylum-seeking process – requiring them to demonstrate a 'well-founded fear of persecution' in line with the requirements of the 1951 UNHCR Refugee Convention. Most children do not receive refugee status as a result, but are instead given time-limited protections and support in the UK for the duration of their childhood. Depending on the age at which they arrive and, given the notoriously lengthy procedures in determining the outcome of claims for asylum, by the time they receive a decision from the Home Office, on or after their eighteenth birthday, many have spent a number of their formative years in Britain. During this time they build friendships and networks, a sense of belonging and have begun to imagine futures in the UK, based around their new experiences of education, aspirations and world-views. If they are not granted the right to remain in the UK, turning 18 for many can mean a sudden change in status, including the complete removal of all forms of support, immediate destitution, the prospect of detention and imminent return to countries of origin, or being forced to live illegally in order to avoid deportation.

It has been argued elsewhere that there is compelling evidence that a sense of wellbeing for children and young people migrating alone to the UK is intrinsically linked to their being able to establish a sense of routine, predictability and stability in their lives – that is, a sense of ontological security (Chase 2013). While the turmoil encountered prior to and during transit to the UK frequently threatens the core of their identity and leaves them feeling fundamentally insecure, given opportunities and resources, young people often find ways to build or regain feelings of security. Such resources are variously derived through friendships, social networks, support from civil society organisations, or faith in God and/or religion. Ultimately, however, the fundamental building blocks of ontological security, and the resources required to enable young people to have a sense of who they are and who they might become, are specific rights and entitlements and thus speak directly to issues of justice.

Broadly speaking, there exist five domains of rights relevant to migrant children and young people who arrive on their own in the UK and then make the transition to adulthood: their (potential) rights as refugees; their rights as children; their rights as looked-after children and young people (and subsequently care leavers); their rights as non-citizens with legitimate temporary status in the UK; and their rights as humans.

The asylum-seeking process is founded on a very particular set of legal procedures which mean that access to due processes of justice is critical in determining the outcomes for young people. Soon after arrival in the UK, children complete a statement of evidence form in the presence of a solicitor, detailing the events leading up to their forced departure from their country of origin, their journey to the UK and what they perceive would be the consequences of returning. This 'interview' is often conducted through an interpreter and usually (but not always) takes place in the presence of a social work professional or foster carer. Subsequently, and prior to their eighteenth birthday, every young person who has not been given a right to remain in the UK in accordance with the refugee convention, has to make a legal case as to why they should be allowed to remain for an extended period of time. There is evidence that they are increasingly likely to have these claims refused (Refugee Council 2017). If this happens, there are situations in which it is possible to make an appeal against the decision or it may be possible to make a fresh claim for asylum (for example as a result of new evidence coming to light regarding their asylum claim). The bureaucratic technicalities of these procedures require expert professional legal advice and guidance.

The reflections included in this chapter emerge from a substantive body of work spanning more than a decade which has explored the wellbeing outcomes of unaccompanied migrant children and young people subject to immigration control in the UK. The first study (2006–07), funded by the Department of Health in England, examined the factors influencing the emotional health and wellbeing of unaccompanied children and young people seeking asylum in the UK (Chase *et al.* 2008). The subsequent 'In Protracted Limbo' study (2012–13), funded by the Oxford University Fell-Fund (Chase and Allsopp 2013, Allsopp and Chase 2014), was a scoping study which culminated in a successful proposal for a three-year ESRC[1] research project entitled 'Becoming Adult' (2016–18), which investigated the wellbeing outcomes of former unaccompanied migrant young people transitioning to adulthood with varied legal status (Chase and Allsopp forthcoming 2019, www.becomingadult.net).

Drawing on a sociology of rights, this chapter considers the practice of justice through the lived experiences of unaccompanied migrant young people and particularly at the point of coming of age in the UK. Issues of access to and equity of 'justice' are fundamental to how young people experience this juncture in their lives. The chapter considers some of the complex facilitators and barriers to young people's access to justice across multiple spheres of their lives and how these combine to magnify elements of chance and serendipity in determining their wellbeing outcomes.

A sociological discourse of rights and justice

At the heart of a genuinely sociological discourse of rights and social justice are three key questions: first, to what extent are rights or, for our purposes, social justice, universally attainable; second, what is the difference between human rights and justice contained within legislative frameworks and a concept of human rights which is grounded in moral obligations and reciprocity; and third, what are the social processes which in practice mediate people's access to rights and justice?

The discourse of legal rights has evolved over many decades and is historically grounded in property rights, generating increasingly sophisticated systems with which to arbitrate the proper allocation of goods and privileges. By contrast, a sociological framing of rights and justice has only come more recently to the stage (see for example Turner 1993, Douzinas 2000, 2009a, 2009b, 2009c, Freeman 2002a, 2002b, Woodiwiss 2005, Benton 2006, Landman 2006, Morris 2006, 2009). While the legal discourse of rights is concerned with the letter of the law and the arbitration through the courts of who has access to what, a sociological analysis of rights applies an inherently normative and moral lens. It asks questions such as whether rights and privileges are just, whether they are fairly administered, whose interests they protect, how rights come into social being and how they operate in social practice (Morris 2006).

These moral dimensions of rights are born out of a classical view of natural law and natural rights from the seventeenth and eighteenth centuries. The classical view held that all individuals within a given society have an inherent sense of justice – people, if left to their own devices, will act in ways towards each other which are conducive to allowing individuals to exercise their fundamental freedoms. Benton (2006) recognises two 'moral intuitions' (p. 21) in this classical discourse of rights: 'the moral priority accorded to the well-being of the individual person, and the notion that all individuals have equal value, are equally worthy of respectful treatment'.

The United States Declaration of Independence (1776) and the French Declaration of the Rights of Man and Citizen (1789) – the precursors of the concept of universal rights – brought with them the imposition of legal order which would guarantee the rights of individuals to freedom, provided that these individuals did not interfere or restrict the freedom of others. If governments failed to uphold or violated certain inalienable rights (such as life, liberty and the pursuit of happiness in the USA; or liberty, property, security and resistance to oppression in France), the citizens of the state had the right to abolish the government. From then on, individuals (in these countries at least) were said to be protected from restrictions to their freedom through a legal order. Yet such rights met with scepticism from philosophers such as Marx and Weber for being bourgeois and exclusionary and inextricably linked to processes of dominance, power and status. Far from being universal, they are largely unattainable to people living in poverty, to the stateless and to women, among others.

Turner (1993) offered the first outline of a sociology of rights around three analytical props: 'ontological frailty'; 'social precariousness'; and 'moral sympathy' (p. 489). Ontological or embodied frailty, Turner claimed, was a human universal condition, compounded by the risky and precarious nature of social institutions. Such vulnerability could therefore be mitigated by an institution of rights, which protects human beings from ontological uncertainty. The efficacy of such an institution, however, was contingent on there being a 'collective sympathy' and therefore had an intrinsically moral character.

Turner's theory of ontological frailty as a universalising concept is especially relevant to the issue of migrant young people's claims to resources which might secure them a viable future. Turner sees a dynamic relationship between human vulnerability and the precarious character of social institutions. All human beings are therefore ontologically members of a community of suffering; 'human frailty is a universal feature of human existence' (Turner 1993, p. 504). And with this frailty comes the possibility for collective or moral sympathy – people have an awareness of their own frailty and so the strong can empathise with the weak, something which Douzinas (2009b) refers to as the pursuit of a shared universal moral code.

From a sociological perspective, therefore, the notions of collective sympathy and a shared moral code provide the fundamental bases for the institution of rights and justice. Applying these concepts to the lived experiences of unaccompanied migrant children transitioning to 'adulthood' in the UK enables us to interrogate the range of moral positionings which come into play in determining young people's outcomes.

The multiple arbiters of social justice

Sometimes I wonder you know. Sometimes people come here and they are too lucky. They have everything and sometimes people they come here and have nothing at all.

The above quotation, which comes from a young woman who participated in the first of the studies cited earlier, neatly captures the perception of chance. What or who determines who gets what, why some young people can stay and others are forced to leave? Cumulative research experience across the past decade clearly indicates that there is no logical system or structure to explain these different outcomes, but something far less tangible and complex is at play. In order to try and make sense of young people's experiences of accessing rights and justice in the context of migrating alone, I pick up the earlier points about human frailty and collective sympathy and consider how they play out through the multi-layered systems and structures which ultimately determine young people's outcomes.

The nation state

At the level of the nation state, a number of social practices determine the actual access to rights and justice (Arendt 1951, Morris 2006, 2009). In practice, rights become enmeshed in political debates concerning whose interests and entitlements should take priority over others. Rather than being constant and universal, rights are therefore in a persistent state of flux. Constituting a permanent work in progress, and determined by different norms and practices of judgement (Freeman 2002a), rights are in effect socially constructed.

There are numerous contemporary examples of how socially constructed rights sustain those with most power and undermine the needs of others who may be disadvantaged as a result of factors such as their gender, ethnicity, sexual identity, ability, age or citizenship status. Recent UK history has witnessed the rise in anti-migration sentiments (exemplified by the decision to leave the European Union following a national referendum in 2016) and media-fuelled moral panic about the numbers of people arriving in the UK. Efforts by the government to regain public support have resulted in more and more stringent asylum and immigration policies – typified by an explicit policy objective of creating a 'hostile environment' in the form of an increasingly punitive immigration and asylum context in the UK, and one which reflects broader trends across Europe (see for example Marfleet 2006, Heuser 2008, Düvell 2009, Squire 2009, Baldwin-Edwards et al. 2018).

Preventing people from specific countries from seeking asylum, criminalising those who fail to claim asylum within a limited time period or who have inadequate documentation, the increased use of welfare restrictions as a means to enforce immigration controls, and increased surveillance through fingerprinting, monitoring and identity cards (McDonald and Bellings 2007, ILPA 2007, 2009) are all indicative of this trend. Moreover, the increasing devolution of immigration controls to education, health and social care institutions (Yuval-Davis et al. 2017) means that immigration control has become everybody's business and is no longer the sole domain of the UK Home Office. Taken together, these measures amount to the contraction of individual and collective rights of those seeking asylum and set the political landscape for the treatment of children and young people subject to immigration control.

At the same time, the hostile environment has simultaneously formulated in the public imagination the stereotypical 'migrant' who scams the system, takes up disproportionate amounts of social housing, medical and social services, and threatens the jobs and security of British citizens. Moreover, interchangeable terminology and tropes such as 'asylum seeker', 'migrant' and 'illegal immigrant' are at the heart of a largely xenophobic public discourse which tends to construct everyone from outside as either a threat or otherwise undesirable. The dominant representation of the asylum seeker, therefore, further limits their rights – to dignity, to respect, to freedom from discrimination – and thus perpetuates a process which, contrary to upholding human rights, essentially dehumanises. The centrality of the nation state in being both *guarantor* and *transgressor* of human rights (Morris 2006, p. 14) cannot therefore be underestimated.

Day-to-day access to justice

Beyond national-level discourses of immigration and asylum, migrant young people's access to rights and justice is also stratified in an infinite number of other complex and dynamic ways from the moment they enter the country. In order to exercise rights as potential refugees, young people require the assistance of lawyers who believe them; interpreters who do justice to their accounts of what happened to them; immigration officials who are empathetic and allow them to speak about what has happened; and sometimes medical specialists who will attest to them being the age they claim to be or confirm the extent of the trauma they have endured. Hence, in order to exercise their rights as children, young people in the first instance need to be believed by immigration officials and social services employees.

Later, children need access to carers, social workers, key workers, teachers, tutors, GPs, and so on, who are sympathetic and empathetic. They may also require advocacy services or other civic society organisations to intervene on their behalf when they are not recognised as children, a common experience typified by age assessments and disputes (see Crawley 2007). Young people's rights as looked-after children and care leavers are contingent on their being accommodated within local authorities with social services departments adequately resourced to support them, and social workers who are compassionate towards them and who prioritise their needs, rather than those of the institution. They frequently also require the intervention of solicitors, civil society organisations, or other significant others to intervene when their rights and entitlements are contested.

Local authority social services departments are charged with the provision of welfare and support to migrant children and young people and should in principle be well placed to facilitate their access to other resources they require. Yet such departments increasingly have limited resources and capacity to provide such services and a lottery emerges regarding access and quality of care for unaccompanied migrant children and young people across different geographic areas (Humphris and Sigona 2017). Furthermore, as argued elsewhere (Chase *et al.* 2008, Chase 2010), professionals are increasingly conflicted in the roles they are expected to play in terms of both supporting young people and having a legal obligation to assist in the control of borders, hence undermining the fundamental rights-based principles of the social work code of practice (Humphries 2004, 2016). The net result is that social care practitioners working with unaccompanied young people are forced to draw distinctions between who they will and will not provide assistance to, and in what ways. Because of this, they must assume a moral stance in relation to individual young people and form judgements as to who are the deserving and who are undeserving of support.

While legal aid services and civil society advocacy organisations are better placed to independently uphold the rights of all children and young people with respect to the letter of the law, they are similarly constrained in what they can and cannot do through systematic restrictions to their resources and funding by successive governments.

Ultimately the decision as to whether or not a young person is granted a right to remain is made by a Home Office official, who may never meet the young person. The arbitrary nature of this decision-making is well known among those who work with refugee and asylum-seeking communities. There is growing evidence that the lottery of the asylum-granting process may to some extent result from the increasing devolution of decision-making powers for individual asylum cases to a range of intermediate actors, including local authority employees. As a number of researchers have observed, this process affords a high degree of discretion and power to an expanding number of individuals and increases the likelihood of subjective and discriminatory decision-making and treatment of asylum seekers which may not necessarily be based on relevant criteria (Holzer *et al.* 2000, Thomas 2006, Camp-Keith and Holmes 2009, Gill 2009). Each of these intermediaries has to make decisions on what constitutes a 'credible' claim for asylum. Thomas (2006) for example has noted how such 'credibility' in asylum claims is culturally bound and quotes one member of Parliament as stating that 'credibility is a way by which the interviewer is able to express his ignorance of the world. What he finds incredible is what surprises him' (Hansard HL Deb., vol. 659, col. 1681,

5 April 2004, cited in Thomas 2006). More recent work by Burridge and Gill (2016) and Gill *et al.* (2018) has highlighted the uneven geographies in access to justice for asylum seekers through legal aid and the chance and luck elements involved in the process and decisions surrounding their asylum claims.

Collective sympathy or antipathy

Throughout the body of research reflected on in this chapter, unaccompanied migrant children and young people have repeatedly described huge differences in how people treated and responded to them at each stage of their encounters with institutional structures and systems relevant to their pursuit of justice. When they first arrived and found themselves embroiled in the asylum claim system, they variously described some people they met as 'nasty' and 'horrible'; and others who demonstrated compassion or care and who intervened on their behalf, even if this was just to ensure that they were able to have food or water. At different stages of the asylum and appeals processes, or in relation to their access to entitlements to social care, housing, education or financial support, young people repeatedly mentioned occasions on which they were unable to exercise certain rights or were at risk of having their rights denied. At these points, it was often the intervention of key individuals or services who mediated on their behalf and facilitated their access to justice and/or core services such as accommodation or financial assistance. Some young people's situations have become causes célèbres due to advocacy efforts involving whole communities, exemplifying the collective moral sympathy alluded to by Turner. One young person in the Becoming Adult project, for example, spoke of how he was on the point of being forcibly removed to Afghanistan when a local media campaign got national attention and the Home Office intervened to release him. Soon after, he was granted indefinite leave to remain in the UK. His reflections on what happened capture the notions of both collective sympathy and antipathy:

> I know there are a lot of good people. You know when I was detained, 3,000 people signed the petition. I never judge everybody by one person ... But some people, you know like I couldn't go forward (with his life) for 10 years. At that time, I couldn't say hello to the police man, now I can say 'hello officer' – but I am the same person. And all this time H (friend) is still here, he signed the petition and called me when I was in the detention centre. That's what you call human, you know? Humans should take care of humans. And you know, sometimes animals take care of each other and the human beings are very useless.

The gatekeepers governing young people's access to justice constitute an incongruous mix of bureaucrats, professionals and caring individuals – some who seemingly make it very difficult for young people to access the support they need, while others work tirelessly to facilitate their access to it. They include politicians and public servants, UK Home Office officials, immigration officers, solicitors, interpreters, foster carers, social workers, teachers/tutors, key workers, personal advisors, psychologists and other health professionals. They also include advocacy services, children's rights organisations, other civil society organisations and individual MPs – the list is endless. They adopt a range of positions in relation to rights and justice at individual as well as institutional levels. Some represent the institutional goals of their organisations such as to control borders or rationalise services, while others (even sometimes within the same institutions) may instead assume a moral position which champions social justice and the rights of others. Equally these different protagonists assume a stance in relation to each migrant young person. Whether they classify a young person, for example, as 'deserving', 'credible' and 'sincere' rather than 'undeserving', devious or, as has emerged frequently throughout the research, not acting as they 'should', fundamentally determines the degree of collective sympathy (Turner 1993) that a young person can muster and which ultimately dictates the extent to which justice is brought within their reach. These different stances are exemplified in the following account from a young man participating in the Department of Health-funded study (Chase *et al.* 2008), although it should be noted that, on some occasions, other young people reported their social worker being their main source of support rather than their adversary:

> The social worker came to see me and she said, 'he is not 15'. I told her that the Home Office believed me and have given me five years, so you can't say that to me. Maybe she didn't like me. Why can she say that? She doesn't even know me. She kept saying, 'he is not 15'. The interpreter said, 'why are you saying that, he is just 15. He is shy and he's really scared – he just came yesterday. How can you say that?' Then they complained about the interpreter. The interpreter never came to see me again, but he just wanted to help me.

Increasingly remote and uncaring asylum systems

If access to justice is based on moral claims and the ability to draw on the sensibilities of a shared understanding of frailty, where does that leave the practice of justice in the context of the 'hostile environment' which has been purposefully generated to deter people from moving to the UK? Moreover, how can such interactions occur when those governing access to justice are increasingly distanced from those who are trying to exercise their right to it?

As implied by Bauman (2004, 2007), the systemised bureaucracy of late modernity and its inherent functional division of labour tends to suppress morality and encourages people to prioritise the purposes of the state over personal wellbeing and the good of others. In the case of young people seeking asylum, this form of bureaucracy is typified by asylum officials making decisions on cases of young people they may never meet and to whom they have no personal or emotional investment; thus there is both practical and mental distance placed between the system determining asylum outcomes and those affected by the decisions. Young people repeatedly talk of how they feel reduced to being a number, that there is no interest in them as a person – and how they view the systems and structures of asylum and immigration as processes of total control. One young woman in the Department of Health-funded study (2006–07) reflected on the arbitrary nature of decision-making about asylum cases and described her efforts to cease being a number and to make sure that she became recognised as an individual through persistently writing to the Home Office:

> I am thinking that someone in the Home Office as we speak now, someone who is working in the Home Office – I am sure they are not seated with their feet up. There is someone out there wearing glasses, really trying to concentrate on someone's case … trying to decide what to do next. I try to think like what they are doing in that time and I am thinking they are doing a lot. And they say they have something like 60,000 cases at one time. And I can just imagine how many documents they have to go through. And I am thinking to myself, 'my document is somewhere in there'. But if I can put in a reminder, constantly pressure them … my case is going to stand out … it is not just going to be put under there. Someone is going to say, 'this person has been writing too much, can someone take her case and review it?' I don't want to be that person who is waiting for six, eight years … 'cos I am not comfortable. I feel like something has to be done. I need to be told where I stand, you know, because I really don't know.

Discussion and conclusion

As discussed earlier, migrant young people arriving alone in the UK have access to five domains of potential rights as they make the transition to adulthood: their (potential) rights as refugees; their rights as children; their rights as looked-after children and young people (and subsequently care leavers); their rights as non-citizens with legitimate temporary status in the UK; and their rights as humans.

If, by the time they turn 18, young people have no legal right to remain in the UK, they enter early 'adulthood' with few, highly contingent rights. At this transition, they face the potential end to discretionary leave (granted according to their status as 'children'); have commonly exhausted the appeals process and hence have no further access to legal processes; no longer meet the criteria of 'children' with respect to international frameworks such as the United Nations Convention on the Rights of the Child (UNCRC); and frequently face substantially fewer rights as care leavers compared with their looked-after peers who are UK citizens. As they become non-citizen adults, opportunities for contesting their denial of rights are diminished. Ultimately, their claim to the final domain of rights, or 'human rights', risks being devoid of meaning since they have such tentative links to any systems or structures which can uphold their rights as human beings. At this juncture, therefore, they risk becoming both state-less and rights-less.

However, the converse scenario is equally possible. There are examples throughout the body of research described here demonstrating that when different people acted either on their own or collectively to lobby on behalf of young people, things did happen and things did change for the better. Practical justice then became something tangible with sometimes transformative results. A recently published short animation entitled *Dear Habib*, and produced for the Becoming Adult project (available at: https://becomingadult.net/) captures beautifully the story of one migrant young person while reflecting the anxieties and dilemmas for many others. It does this by telling Habib's story, the distress and trauma he experiences throughout his migration, the strength of the relationships he builds and how these fundamentally determine what happens to him. What Habib's story illustrates best are both the human frailty generated by life circumstances and events, and the ad hoc acts of human kindness and 'collective sympathy' which ultimately provide him with a pathway to build his life and future here in the UK.

Young people interviewed throughout the research described in this same project were acutely aware of the extent of luck and lack of logic in how decisions on asylum claims were made. Several talked of how they could not understand why others they knew had been granted indefinite leave to remain with apparently weaker claims to asylum than themselves. On the other hand, others knew of young people who had been refused and in some cases returned to countries of origin, and they felt 'bad' that these young people had not had the same opportunities as themselves. One young man from the Becoming Adult project who had secured legal status in the UK after seven years commented on the difficulty of managing conversations with friends who had spent their youth in the UK but who nonetheless had been deported:

> When he calls he asks, 'how is X (the name of the city)?, how is it doing?' Or, 'What about this person, how is he doing?', or 'Do you remember when we barbecued in this place?', and 'Do you remember those pictures?', and 'Have you got those pictures?' And stuff like that.

And sometimes you feel like you don't want to talk about it because you will upset the person, isn't it? But you feel like you are lucky because you are still here, but you feel sorry about the person who didn't get to stay.

The arguments presented in this chapter draw strength from the depth and longevity of the evidence at hand. Many of the difficulties related to young people's transition to 'adulthood' emerged in the first Department of Health-funded study (2006–07) even though it was not the primary focus of the research. In particular the evident arbitrariness of whether young people could access services, support and legal advice and justice came very much to the fore. Ten years on, as I write up the findings from the most recent ESRC-supported Becoming Adult study, the insights from a justice perspective are strikingly similar. There is no logic to the likelihood of receiving refugee status; there is no systematic access to justice or legal recourse for making a claim to stay in the UK; there is no pattern in the likelihood that the social worker, foster carer or teacher with whom a young person builds a relationship will be in a position or take the moral stance to mediate and support their access to justice and rights in ways which bring about a positive outcome. As such, serendipity and chance combined with moral judgements are as likely to determine the outcomes for young people as any process of legal rights or justice.

The theatre of rights and justice is evidently played out on many different stages. Whether these be supra-national, national, local or individual dramas, they continue to raise fundamental questions about the universality of rights and their relevance to the plight of individuals. While I have considered the various ways in which the UK asylum and immigration system upholds or withholds rights and the various posturing that takes place (see for example Landman 2006), it is at the micro-level analysis of the factors influencing individuals' access to rights and justice that we see the propensity for luck and serendipity.

An adequate theory of practical justice needs to recognise the multiple arbiters of social justice and the powerful roles they can assume in simultaneously widening access to it for some while closing its doors to others. For the young people who were part of this body of research over a substantial period of time, the patterns of serendipity and chance appear paradoxically consistent. As a result, migrant young people continue to struggle with how they might navigate their way to the futures they aspire to with no clear signs or signals to guide them, and no evident rules to the social justice game.

Note

1 The Economic and Social Research Council (ESRC) is one of the major funding bodies for the social sciences in the UK.

References

Allsopp, A. and Chase, E., 2014. The Tactics of Time and Status: Young People's Experiences of Building Futures While Subject to Immigration Control in Britain. *Journal of Refugee Studies*, 28 (2), 163–182.

Arendt, H., 1951. *The Origins of Totalitarianism*. New York: Harcourt Brace.

Baldwin-Edwards, M., Blitz, B. and Crawley, H., eds, 2018. *Journal of Ethnic and Migration Studies*. Special Issue: The European Union in Crisis: A collective failure to protect refugees and migrants.

Bauman, Z., 2004. *Wasted Lives: Modernity and its Outcasts*. Cambridge: Polity Press.

Bauman, Z., 2007. *Liquid Times: Living in an Age of Uncertainty*. Cambridge: Polity Press.

Benton, T., 2006. Do We Need Rights? If So, What Sort? In: L. Morris, ed., *Rights: Sociological Perspectives*. Abingdon: Routledge, 21–36.

Burridge, A. and Gill, N., 2016. Conveyor-Belt Justice: Precarity, Access to Justice, and Uneven Geographies of Legal Aid in UK Asylum Appeals. *Antipode*, 49 (1), 23–42.

Camp-Keith, L. and Holmes, J., 2009. A Rare Examination of Typically Unobservable Factors in US Asylum Decisions. *Journal of Refugee Studies*, 22 (2), 224–241.

Chase, E., 2010. Agency and Silence: Young People Seeking Asylum Alone in the UK. *British Journal of Social Work*, 40 (7), 2050–2068.

Chase, E., 2013. Security and Subjective Wellbeing: The Experiences of Unaccompanied Young People Seeking Asylum in the UK. *Sociology of Health and Illness*, 35 (6), 358–372.

Chase, E. and Allsopp, J., 2013. 'Future Citizens of the World'?: The Contested Futures of Independent Young Migrants in Europe. RSC Working Papers Series, 97. Oxford: Refugee Studies Centre.

Chase, E. and Allsopp, J., forthcoming, 2019. *The Politics of Wellbeing in Transition*. Bristol: Policy Press.

Chase, E., Knight, A. and Statham, J., 2008. *The Emotional Wellbeing of Unaccompanied Young People Seeking Asylum in the UK*. London: BAAF.

Crawley, H., 2007. *When is a Child not a Child? Asylum, Age Disputes and the Process of Age Assessments*. London: ILPA.

Douzinas, C., 2000. *The End of Human Rights: Critical Legal Thought at the Turn of the Century*. Oxford: Hart Publishing.

Douzinas, C., 2009a. Are Rights Universal? *Guardian*, 11 March.

Douzinas, C., 2009b. What Are Human Rights? *Guardian*, 18 March.

Douzinas, C., 2009c. Who Counts as Human? *Guardian*, 1 April.

Düvell, F., 2009. *Irregular Migration in Northern Europe: Overview and Comparison*. Paper given at Clandestino Project Conference. London, 27 March.

Freeman, M., 2002a. *Human Rights: An Interdisciplinary Approach*. Cambridge: Polity Press, and Oxford: Blackwell Publishers Ltd.

Freeman, M., 2002b. Human Rights, Children's Rights and Judgement – Some Thoughts on Reconciling Universality and Pluralism. *International Journal of Children's Rights*, 10, 345–354.

Gill, N., 2009. Presentational State Power: Temporal and Spatial Influences over Asylum Sector Decision Makers. *Transactions of the Institute of British Geographers*, 34 (2), 215–233.

Gill, N., Rotter, R., Burridge, A. and Allsopp, J., 2018. The Limits of Procedural Discretion: Unequal Treatment and Vulnerability in Britain's Asylum Appeals. *Social and Legal Studies*, 27 (1), 49–78.

Heuser, S., 2008. Is There a Right to Have Rights? The Case of the Right to Asylum. *Ethical Theory and Moral Practice*, 11 (1), 3–13.

Holzer, T., Schneider, G. and Widmer, T., 2000. Federalism and the Handling of Asylum Applications in Switzerland, 1988–1996. *Journal of Conflict Resolution*, 44 (2), 250–276.

Humphries, B., 2004. An Unacceptable Role for Social Work: Implementing Immigration Policy. *British Journal of Social Work*, 34, 93–107.

Humphries, B., 2016. Taking Sides: Social Work Research as a Moral and Political Activity. In: R. Lovelock, K. Lyons and J. Powell, eds, *Reflecting on Social Work: Discipline and Profession*. Farnham: Ashgate Publishing, 113–130.

Humphris, R. and Sigona, N., 2017. Outsourcing the 'Best Interests' of Unaccompanied Asylum-seeking Children in the Era of Austerity. *Journal of Ethnicity and Migration*. https://doi.org/10.1080/1369183x.2017.1404266.

ILPA, 2007. *Children's Asylum Claims*. Information Sheet, 5 April. Available from: www.ilpa.org.uk/infoservice.html [Accessed 4 July 2018].

ILPA, 2009. *Joint Committee on Human Rights: Inquiry on Children's Rights: Submission of the Immigration Law Practitioners' Association*. Available from: www.ilpa.org.uk [Accessed 5 July 2018].

Landman, T., 2006. *Studying Human Rights*. London: Routledge.

Marfleet, P., 2006. *Refugees in a Global Era*. Basingstoke: Palgrave Macmillan.

McDonald, I. and Bellings, P., 2007. The Treatment of Asylum Seekers in the UK. *Journal of Social Welfare and Family Law*, 29 (1), 49–65.

Morris, L., ed., 2006. *Rights: Sociological Perspectives*. Abingdon: Routledge.

Morris, L., 2009. Civic Stratification and the Cosmopolitan Ideal. *European Societies*, 11 (4), 603–624.

Refugee Council, 2017. *Children in the Asylum System*. Available from: www.refugeecouncil.org.uk/assets/0004/2380/Children_in_the_Asylum_System_Nov_2017.pdf.

Squire, V., 2009. *The Exclusionary Politics of Asylum*. Basingstoke: Palgrave Macmillan.

Thomas, R., 2006. Assessing the Credibility of Asylum Claims: EU and UK Approaches Examined. *European Journal of Migration and Law*, 8, 1, 79–96.

Turner, B., 1993. Outline of a Theory of Human Rights. *Sociology*, 27 (3), 489–512.

Woodiwiss, A., 2005. *Human Rights*. Key Ideas series. London: Routledge.

Yuval-Davis, N., Wemyss, G. and Cassidy, K. 2017. Everyday Bordering, Belonging and the Re-orientation of British Immigration Legislation. *Sociology*, 52, 2, 228–244.

Chapter 13

Patient-reported measures as a justice project through involvement of service-user researchers

Annie Madden, Paul Lennon, Cassie Hogan, Mel Getty, Max Hopwood, Joanne Neale and Carla Treloar

Introduction

There is growing interest in the development of patient-reported measures in the health care sector as a means to improving the quality of services provided (Chen *et al.* 2013, Nelson *et al.* 2015, Greenhalgh *et al.* 2017). However, there is a key foundational aspect on which approaches to the development and use of patient-reported measures differ; namely, in the extent to which service users have been involved in the development of the measure. Diana Rose (2014) has previously described the ethical imperative of public involvement in research, particularly for social marginalised groups, because 'changing the knowledge producers will change the knowledge itself' (p. 149). In recognition of this, Rose and colleagues (2011) proposed a new method for developing patient-reported measures that involve service-user researchers at all stages. They argued that this is necessary as people who use services may have very different perspectives on what constitutes a positive treatment experience or health-related outcome compared with the perspectives of those who provide the services or conduct research within related fields.

As a group of researchers in the UK and Australia, we have been much involved in developing patient-reported measures for people with experience of alcohol and other drug use. The approach our work has taken has viewed the experience and expertise of service users as central to the development of the new measures. As part of this work, we have developed research projects on issues as diverse as recovery from alcohol and other drug use, sleep among those who use alcohol and other drugs, and the experience and outcomes of hepatitis C treatment for people who inject drugs. Each project used a qualitative approach to develop domains and candidate items for potential inclusion in a new instrument to measure the factors that service users viewed as important. The instruments developed by a team at King's College London (see Table 13.1) to measure recovery and sleep relied on frequent input from an expert Service User Research Group (represented here by PL, CH and MG). The team in Sydney, which is developing measures for hepatitis C treatment

Table 13.1 Patient-reported measures

The instruments that our work has developed include:

1 Recovery – for recovery from drug and alcohol dependence, Substance Use Recovery Evaluator (SURE) (Neale, Vitoratou *et al.* 2016)

2 Sleep – to assess sleep amongst people experiencing problems with alcohol or other drugs, the Substance Use Sleep Scale (SUSS) (Neale *et al.* 2018)

3 Experience and outcomes of direct-acting antiviral treatment of hepatitis for people who inject drugs (Madden *et al.* forthcoming)

---

for people who inject drugs, included a peer researcher (AM) who was involved in all aspects of the research. The London and Sydney models of service-user involvement are different in terms of structure and process, but share an important key element: the explicit acknowledgement and valuing of knowledge and expertise based in lived experience.

This chapter focuses on what justice might mean in the practice of developing and implementing patient-reported measures for people with experience of alcohol and other drug services. The content of this chapter derives from team discussions occurring in London and Sydney, as well as from individual self-reflection. Throughout, the views of the service users involved in research development and implementation are foregrounded.

Why service-user involvement is needed when developing patient-reported measures for people who use alcohol and other drugs

Involving services users in the development of patient-reported measures can have instrumental benefits while also addressing macro issues of power imbalances and stigma towards people who use alcohol and other drugs. At the instrumental level, researchers can learn how to make their measures 'better'. While some researchers will have experience of using or being dependent on alcohol or other drugs, they are likely to be in the minority and even fewer will have had direct experience of injecting drug use. Involving service users in the process of developing patient-reported measures can help researchers assess if the questions they are asking are likely to be interpreted in the ways they want them to be interpreted by the target population; and this is particularly important when developing new measures. Indeed, this speaks directly to the issue of validity: are the measures, and items within them, going to capture what the study is aiming for? Overlaying this is, of course, the social distance that often exists between people who use alcohol and other drug services and the people who conduct research within them – a distance that can be compounded by the stigma, discrimination and criminality often associated with the use of illicit substances.

In order to learn or benefit from service-user involvement in the development of patient-reported measures, researchers need to acknowledge the
power dynamics at play within the research process. Power, stigma and
discrimination can result in service users feeling deeply disenfranchised and
disempowered. Often people who use illicit drugs have little sense of entitlement to the health system because they are widely understood to be 'socially
irresponsible people' and therefore undeserving of access to healthcare. Such
attitudes result in people being 'dismissed' when attempting to engage with
health services and/or poorly treated if they do gain access. Accordingly, they
may have few 'hopes and dreams' for their health or their future, or only
hope that their health might not get worse. Academic researchers may
struggle to appreciate the extent to which these feelings can profoundly affect
people's lives and the decisions that people who use alcohol and other drugs
make about their health. Researchers may consequently overlook or discount
these issues when trying to measure or account for the experiences of service
users. Involving people with lived experience in development of patient-
reported measures can illuminate what is really important and, in so doing,
highlight and then begin to challenge the effects of health-related stigma and
the power imbalances which facilitate stigma.

Stigma may also manifest itself in interactions between researchers and
service users engaged in research. Service users who are engaged in
research processes are sometimes looked down upon and discredited by
researchers. The experience of researchers consulting with service users as
equals with the common goal of improving services may help to challenge
negative stereotypical views and reduce the stigmatisation of people who
use alcohol and other drugs. In turn, this can have other benefits.

In general terms, researchers occupy powerful positions as custodians
of knowledge-generation and dissemination. Service users may be interested in being part of research groups, such as a service user research
group, or engaged in research in other ways, because doing so offers
opportunities to advance government policy for alcohol and other drug
treatment, and influence how drug dependence is seen in a political
context. In this way, service-user involvement in development of patient-
reported measures, and in research more generally, is a means to be on
the 'ground level' of efforts to have service users' needs clearly represented within research outcomes and to have their concerns and contributions visible to the people in power.

Why is there a need for patient-reported measures in alcohol and other drug services?

Patient-reported measures can help to shape the ways that services are
designed and delivered so that they better meet the needs and preferences
of service users (Black 2013, Basch 2017). A range of factors influence the

design and delivery of services, including budget and policy, and patient-reported measures are based on the premise that these factors should also include the views of the people who are using the service. As power differences, stigma, discrimination and criminality can create particular experiences or expectations of health services, issues that matter to people using alcohol and other drugs are often not reflected in current service provision or assessment of outcomes. The use of a patient-reported measure can 'forge space' where service users and service providers communicate, so providing an opportunity for clinicians to see and value the input of service users.

Developing treatment measures without the involvement of service users can result not only in service users' further disengagement from the health system, but also in promoting harmful attitudes and values among clinicians. This is especially the case when the topic of measurement is complex and difficult to define, such as recovery from drug and alcohol use, leading to reliance on basic indicators, particularly measures of reduced drug use and criminal activity (Neale, Panebianco *et al.* 2016). For example, one key outcome measure used across services in the UK, the Treatment Outcomes Profile, while only brief, includes questions about crimes (shoplifting; selling drugs; theft from or of a vehicle; other property theft or burglary; fraud, forgery, or handling stolen goods; committing assault or violence) (Marsden *et al.* 2008). This is often perceived by service users as 'offensive' as the question, and by implication the whole measure, assumes a link between the use of alcohol and other drugs and crime. The use of this measure therefore 'perpetuates' the well-worn stereotype that 'all drug users are criminals'.

Given the limitations of existing instruments and the growing interest in patient-reported measures across the wider health sector, it is surprising that there has not been greater interest in these measures in the alcohol and other drugs field. Indeed, this is the gap that our work in London and Sydney aims to fill. The term 'recovery' from alcohol and other drug use gained currency in the UK during the early 2000s (HM Government 2010) but research conducted as part of the London patient-reported measure programme (Neale *et al.* 2015) showed how service users and professionals had different views on what constitutes 'recovery' and that professionals can sometimes have little understanding of what service users actually want from services. For example, service providers and service funders can over-prioritise the reduction of drug use, or indeed abstinence, as treatment outcomes; yet, a much wider range of factors are needed to adequately reflect and measure service users' views of progress and success. Measures of progress and success in drug treatment services therefore need to be de-coupled from measures of extent of drug use.

The recovery patient-reported measure does just that. There is little focus on the use of alcohol or other drugs. Progress or success in treatment is instead referred to by domains such as self-care, relationships, material resources and outlook on life. This measure was developed by drawing on qualitative research with service users and research with service providers (Neale *et al.* 2014, Neale, Panebianco *et al.* 2016) and involved members of the service users' research group at each step to provide expert oversight and direction on choice of concepts, wording and measurement options. From personal communications with researchers and practitioners, the recovery patient-reported measure is now being used within many services across the UK and internationally, with Norwegian, Spanish and Italian translations and cultural adaptations available or in progress. A mobile phone app for both SURE and SUSS is currently being planned, again with extensive service-user input.

The recovery and sleep patient-reported measures provided a model for the development of a patient-reported measure for delivery of direct-acting antiviral treatment for hepatitis C among people who inject drugs. The last five years have seen a revolution in hepatitis C treatment. Direct-acting antiviral therapies are highly effective, with a more tolerable side effect profile than previous interferon-based treatments. This advance in treatment has led to global advocacy efforts toward the elimination of hepatitis C (Grebely *et al.* 2013); indeed, the World Health Organization has provided targets for the elimination of hepatitis C by 2030, a public health challenge (World Health Organization 2016).

This focus on elimination led our team to think about the ways in which the priorities of service users were being represented (or not) in this dialogue and in treatment delivery. Our team includes the first author, who has experience as someone who has injected drugs, lived with hepatitis C and been a national and international advocate for the rights of her community. To shape this project we drew on her experience, from discussions with her peers living with hepatitis C and from the clinical and epidemiological literature. As a team, we were concerned that outcomes of treatment 'beyond cure' were virtually absent from the literature and that this would undermine service delivery and evaluation of direct-acting antiviral treatment implementation.

As with alcohol and other treatment and service provision, the ways in which direct-acting antiviral treatments are delivered are shaped by macro forces of power, stigma and criminalisation. Just as alcohol and other drug services may over-prioritise reductions in drug use and abstinence as treatment outcomes, so the focus on elimination seemed likely to draw clinicians and researchers to clinical outcomes (cure), at the expense of other factors, such as the stigma and discredit inherent in the health system or the ways in which the treatment-related concerns of people living with hepatitis C have been systematically downplayed or ignored within health services. In this kind of situation, the development of a hepatitis C treatment patient-reported measure could give voice and legitimacy to people who do not feel entitled to provide feedback to their carers about what is important to them.

To develop the patient-reported measure for hepatitis C treatment, our team worked in a participatory way, with a fully embedded peer researcher (AM). With the assistance of a peer-based drug-user organisation in the Australian state of Victoria, Harm Reduction Victoria, people with histories of injecting drug use and a hepatitis C diagnosis were recruited to participate in interviews about what they valued or expected from treatment for hepatitis C. The team used these interviews to construct draft items for two new measures: a patient-reported experience measure and a patient-reported outcome measure. These draft items were subsequently reviewed in focus groups by a second sample of people with a history of injecting drug use who had received direct-acting antiviral therapy for hepatitis C – again, with the assistance of Harm Reduction Victoria and a second community organisation in the same state, Hepatitis Victoria.

Analyses revealed that hepatitis C treatment should be evaluated by a wide range of factors beyond cure, such as: improvements in physical and mental health; being provided with a plan for ongoing liver health care; confidence in understanding test results; confidence in managing future risk of HCV infection; feeling more positive about life and the future; coping better with daily life and responsibilities; and changes in self-perception and identity. In the interviews with people living with hepatitis C at the start of the study, however, we found that it was difficult to 'get discussion going'. The notion that a person who injects drugs could actually have an opinion of health care seemed to be unfamiliar and unexpected for some people. In the focus groups, where draft instruments were provided for feedback, the conversation flowed more easily. The feedback was very positive, with participants stating that 'no one' had previously asked them what they wanted from treatment and that 'cure' was (too narrowly) the only outcome discussed or anticipated during their treatment.

While the number of people treated for hepatitis C in Australia initially surged following release of publicly subsidised direct-acting antiviral treatments, these numbers have since plateaued (Kirby Institute 2017). In response, there have been calls for more sophisticated approaches to attracting people with hepatitis C and experience of injecting drug use into treatment (Henderson *et al.* 2017). If we explicitly recognise and acknowledge that direct-acting antiviral treatments can offer much more than a cure for hepatitis C, it might encourage more people to come forward for liver health monitoring and health care. Patient-reported measures demonstrate how services can contribute to a diverse range of outcomes, including those justice-related, and are focused on delivering person-centred care; this can potentially make those services more attractive to the people they seek to help or treat.

As we write, the hepatitis C patient-reported measures are in draft form and require testing on larger samples of people experiencing therapy before they have the status of a validated measure. However, these measures have already met some of their goals. As with all of the measures developed by our teams, a key underlying aim was to generate change through the development process. Being on the 'ground floor' can exert influence by highlighting and redefining what gets counted, which is critical in the context of the old maxim of 'what gets counted, counts'. Patient-reported measures can thus instil justice into the health system by changing the framework of service evaluation. The use of a patient-reported measure positions service-user values as central to this framework and, in essence, makes workers and the system accountable for delivering services that support these values. A fundamental aspect of the patient-reported measures discussed in this chapter is the centrality of service-user researchers in the process of developing these instruments. We now turn to a broader discussion of justice in working with service-user researchers.

What does justice mean when working with service-user researchers?

Throughout academia, researchers have not tended to involve people who use alcohol and other drug services in the process of conducted research: instead of being respected partners, they have been positioned as the 'subjects' of enquiry. There are, however, numerous ways that researchers and service users can work together when conducting research (Neale et al. 2017). For example, the service users' research group in London generally offers researchers initial one-off consultations followed by occasional follow-up advice and support. This may be sufficient for some projects and can provide a means of involving people who are currently injecting or using substances or in treatment within the research process. For the London patient-reported measure projects, the service users' research group was more heavily involved, providing repeated input throughout the project. As indicated earlier, the Sydney patient-reported measures project operated differently, again with a peer researcher (AM) embedded in the research team and employed as a university staff member.

Whatever the structure of engagement, a number of key principles are necessary to ensure that research projects are conducted in a just manner. Payment of service-user researchers is one of these, not least because payment 'confers a level of respect'. Service users engaged in research provide 'professional advice' to researchers and this advice should be considered equivalent to 'any other part played in the project' by service users or other researchers. Payment is an acknowledgement of time and expertise and may also be essential when there are material costs (such as transport, childcare or loss of earnings) involved in participation. Researchers can also provide acknowledgement of the input from service users by naming them as co-authors on reports, papers or grant applications, and at the very least by providing feedback on what happened to studies they participated in. Without this, service users may question whether researchers fully 'respected their opinions' by following or incorporating the advice they provided.

The experience for the Sydney project was different in that a peer researcher was part of all decision-making and actions pertaining to the patient-reported measure study. The Sydney team had a commitment to 'practice what we preach' by finding ways for service users to be involved in each step of development of the patient-reported measure. At a broader level, the project posited justice in human rights terms, via the view that service users should be engaged as full citizens in relation to service delivery and in the conduct of research. However, the notion of change and impact were also important as part of this project. The 'measure of the patient-reported measure' (that is, the proof of its value) would lie in what change it could achieve as part of a larger project to promote justice for service users in having their priorities valued by clinicians and service funders.

Conclusion

Our teams have been involved in the development and implementation of patient-reported measures not only as a means to advance scientific understanding of treatment, but as justice projects. The involvement of service users in 'building' these measures was a necessary requirement, but the larger project was to foreground the experience and values of service users that may have otherwise never been canvassed or measured. In a field such as alcohol and other drugs, where research and decisions on services and programmes can so easily be hijacked by political or popular agendas (Wodak 1996, Rehm *et al.* 2010), the need for well-designed patient-reported measures to be a part of the evidence base is vitally important to bring justice to service users. While we work with the maxim 'what gets counted, counts' in the patient-reported measure field, we are aware that these measures by themselves will not do all the work. Similarly, our work is guided by 'what counts doesn't always get counted'. The best-designed patient-reported measure cannot alone counter the long history of dismissal, exclusion and discredit experienced by alcohol and other drug service users nor challenge all of the social and structural forces that perpetuate unjust services. However, projects that develop or use patient-reported measures can be seen bringing two worlds (evidence-based medicine and service-user involvement) together to better the experience of people who may have few resources and little power to express and claim their rights.

Acknowledgements

We thank the participants in this study and are grateful for the support of Harm Reduction Victoria and Hepatitis Victoria. The Centre for Social Research in Health at UNSW Sydney is supported by a grant from the Australian Government Department of Health. The views expressed in this chapter are those of the authors alone and are not necessarily those of any of the funders. This project was supported by a seed grant from the PLuS Alliance.

References

Basch, E., 2017. Patient-reported Outcomes – Harnessing Patients' Voices to Improve Clinical Care. *New England Journal of Medicine*, 376 (2), 105–108.

Black, N., 2013. Patient Reported Outcome Measures Could Help Transform Healthcare. *BMJ: British Medical Journal*, 346.

Chen, J., Ou, L. and Hollis, S. J., 2013. A Systematic Review of the Impact of Routine Collection of Patient Reported Outcome Measures on Patients, Providers and Health Organisations in an Oncologic Setting. *BMC Health Services Research*, 13, 211.

Grebely, J., Graham, C. S., Matthews, G. V., Lloyd, A. R. and Dore, G. J., 2013. Elimination of Hepatitis C Virus Infection among People who Inject Drugs through Treatment as Prevention: Feasibility and Future Requirements. *Clinical Infectious Diseases*, 57 (7), 1014–1020.

Greenhalgh, J., Dalkin, S. and Gooding K., 2017. Health Services and Delivery Research. *Functionality and Feedback: A Realist Synthesis of the Collation, Interpretation and Utilisation of Patient-reported Outcome Measures Data to Improve Patient Care.* Southampton, UK: NIHR Journals Library.

Henderson, C., Madden, A. and Kelsall, J., 2017. 'Beyond the Willing & the Waiting': The Role of Peer-based Approaches in Hepatitis C Diagnosis & Treatment. *International Journal of Drug Policy*, 50, 111–115.

HM Government, 2010. *Reducing Demand, Restricting Supply, Building Recovery: Supporting People to Live Drug Free Life.* London: HM Government.

Kirby Institute, 2017. *Monitoring Hepatitis C Treatment Uptake in Australia* (Issue 8, December 2017). Sydney: Kirby Institute, UNSW Sydney.

Madden, A., Hopwood, M., Neale, J. and Treloar, C., forthcoming. Development of Patient Reported Outcome and Experience Measures for Hepatitis C Treatment among People who Inject Drugs. *The Patient.* doi: 10.1007/s40271-018-0332-6.

Marsden, J., Farrell, M., Bradbury, C., Dale-Perera, A., Eastwood, B., Roxburgh, M. and Taylor, S., 2008. Development of the Treatment Outcomes Profile. *Addiction*, 103, 1450–1460.

Neale, J., Finch, E., Marsden, J., Mitcheson, L., Rose, D., Strang, J., Tompkins, C., Wheeler, C. and Wykes, T., 2014. How Should We Measure Addiction Recovery? Analysis of Service Provider Perspectives Using Online Delphi Groups. *Drugs: Education, Prevention and Policy*, 21, 310–323.

Neale, J., Finch, E., Marsden, J., Mitcheson, L., Rose, D., Strang, J., Tompkins, C., Wheeler, C. and Wykes, T., 2015. 'You're All Going to Hate the Word "Recovery" by the End of This': Service Users' Views of Measuring Addiction Recovery. *Drugs: Education, Prevention and Policy*, 22, 26–34.

Neale, J., Getty, M., Bouteloup, A., Hogan, C., Lennon, P., McCusker, M. and Strang, J., 2017. Why We Should Conduct Research in Collaboration with People Who Use Alcohol and Other Drugs. *Addiction*, 112, 2084–2085.

Neale, J., Panebianco, D., Finch, E., Marsden, J., Mitcheson, L., Rose, D., Strang, J. and Wykes, T., 2016. Emerging Consensus on Measuring Addiction Recovery: Findings from a Multi-stakeholder Consultation Exercise. *Drugs: Education, Prevention and Policy*, 23, 31–40.

Neale, J., Vitoratou, S., Finch, E., Lennon, P., Mitcheson, L., Panebianco, D., Rose, D., Strang, J., Wykes, T. and Marsden, J., 2016. Development and Validation of 'SURE': A Patient Reported Outcome Measure (PROM) for Recovery from Drug and Alcohol Dependence. *Drug and Alcohol Dependence*, 165, 159–167.

Neale, J., Vitoratou, S., Lennon, P., Meadows, R., Nettleton, S., Panebianco, D., Strang, J. and Marsden, J., 2018. Development and Early Validation of a Patient Reported Outcome Measure to Assess Sleep Amongst People Experiencing Problems with Alcohol or Other Drugs. *Sleep*, 41 (4), zsy013.

Nelson, E. C., Eftimovska, E., Lind, C., Hager, A., Wasson, J. H. and Lindblad, S., 2015. Patient Reported Outcome Measures in Practice. *BMJ: British Medical Journal*, 350.

Rehm, J., Fisher, B., Hickman, M., Ball, A., Atun, R., Kazatchkine, M., Southwell, M., Fry, C. and Room, R., 2010. Perspectives on Harm Reduction – What Experts Have to Say. In: T. Rhodes and D. Hedrich, eds, *Harm Reduction: Evidence, Impacts and Challenges*. Spain: European Monitoring Centre for Drugs and Drug Addiction, 79–111.

Rose, D., 2014. Patient and Public Involvement in Health Research: Ethical Imperative and/or Radical Challenge? *Journal of Health Psychology*, 19, 149–158.

Rose, D., Evans, J., Sweeney, A. and Wykes, T., 2011. A Model for Developing Outcome Measures from the Perspectives of Mental Health Service Users. *International Review of Psychiatry*, 23, 41–46.

Wodak, A., 1996. When Medical Research is Beholden to Politics. *Medical Journal of Australia*, 164, 649–650.

World Health Organization, 2016. *Combating Hepatitis B and C to Reach Elimination by 2030: Advocacy Brief*. Geneva: World Health Organization.

Chapter 14

Unequal justice: the effect of mass incarceration on children's educational outcomes in the USA

Practical implications for policy and programmes

Leila Morsy

Introduction

The US criminal justice system incarcerates at a rate without equal in the modern world. In the USA today, there are approximately 700 prisoners per 100,000 residents. The next highest rate can be found in Turkmenistan (with approximately 600), followed by El Salvador and Cuba (500 each) and Thailand (450). Among other Western industrialised nations, the United Kingdom (including England and Wales), Spain and Australia have the highest rates of incarceration (150), while others – Canada and France, for example – have rates of around 100 or below (Wagner and Walsh 2016).

These imprisonment rates are not the result of rising crime. Rather, two policies have been mostly responsible. The first has been an increasingly punitive sentencing policy, including prison terms for violent crimes that have increased by nearly 50 per cent since the early 1990s. The second has been a declaration by the US federal and state governments of a 'war on drugs' that has included severe mandatory minimum sentences for drug offences that are generally not considered to involve a direct victim (Blumstein and Beck 1999, Pfaff 2015, Schanzenbach *et al.* 2016). The trend has been exacerbated by the re-imprisonment of released offenders for technical probation violations or for the inability to pay escalating fines and court fees. Absurdly, while released prisoners are in many cases excluded – either formally or informally – from employment in the legal economy, they can be re-imprisoned for violating the terms of release by failing to hold a job (Robles and Dewan 2015).

Young African-American men are no more likely to use or sell drugs than young white men, but they are nearly three times as likely to be arrested for drug use or sale; once arrested, they are more likely to be sentenced; and, once sentenced, their jail or prison terms are 50 per cent longer on average (Makarechi 2015, Schanzenbach *et al.* 2016). African-American drivers are no more likely than white drivers to change lanes

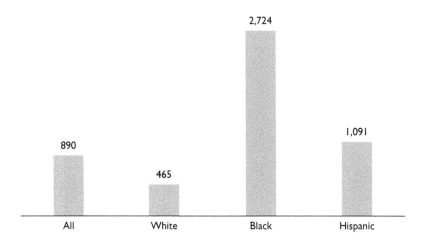

Figure 14.1 Approximate number of men in jail or prison per 100,000 population, by race and ethnicity, 2014.

Source: Bonczar (2003), Carson (2015), Sentencing Project (2017).

without signalling, but they are more likely to be stopped by police for doing so and, once stopped, they are more likely to be caught up in the penal system, including jail time for inability to pay fines (Makarechi 2015, Schanzenbach *et al.* 2016). The US Justice Department's investigation of police practices in Ferguson, Missouri, found that African-Americans were stopped by the police more frequently than whites, but of those who were stopped and searched, more whites were found to be carrying illegal drugs than African-Americans (Makarechi 2015, Schanzenbach *et al.* 2016).

Whites are incarcerated at a rate of approximately 400 per 100,000 white residents, high by international standards but not the highest. The USA's ranking as the nation with the most-incarcerated population is attributable primarily to the imprisonment of 2,200 African-Americans per 100,000 African-American residents, and to a lesser extent to a Hispanic imprisonment rate of nearly 1,000 (Prison Policy Initiative 2016). Figure 14.1 shows the racial and ethnic distribution of incarcerated men (as of 2014) (Bonczar 2003, Carson 2015, Sentencing Project 2017).

Racial and social class differences in children's experiences with parental incarceration

The effects of the tendencies and processes described above are dramatic. By age 14, approximately 25 per cent of African-American children have experienced a parent, in most cases a father, being imprisoned for some period of time. The comparable share for white children is 4 per cent

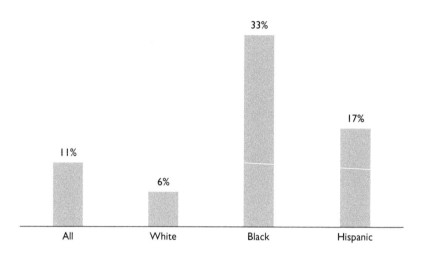

Figure 14.2 Rate of US male imprisonment, by race and ethnicity.
Source: Bonczar (2003), Carson (2015), Sentencing Project (2017).

(Wildeman and Western 2010). On any given school day in 2008, approximately 10 per cent of African-American schoolchildren had a parent in jail or prison, more than four times the share of African-American schoolchildren with a parent in jail or prison in 1980 (Western and Pettit 2010).

This growth in the proportion of African-American children suffering from parental incarceration has in all probability offset many efforts to raise the average achievement levels of these children during the last 35 years. Although the proportion of white children with a father in prison has grown comparably (from 0.5 per cent to 2 per cent), the concentration in low-income neighbourhoods of African-American children with imprisoned fathers presents challenges to teachers and schools unlike those presented by the relatively rare white child with an imprisoned father (Western and Pettit 2010).

Outcomes for children of incarcerated parents

Children of incarcerated parents suffer serious harm, including depressed health and learning outcomes (Foster and Hagan 2009, Geller *et al.* 2009, Johnson 2009, Aaron and Dallaire 2010, Cho 2010, Murray, Loeber and Pardini 2012, Nichols and Loper 2012, Lee *et al.* 2013, Turney 2014, Mears and Siennick 2016). It is tempting to think that these consequences are attributes of the disadvantaged child, independent of parental incarceration. But careful studies of the effects on children have accounted for these attributes. Children of incarcerated parents have worse cognitive and non-cognitive outcomes than children with similar socioeconomic and demographic characteristics whose parents have not experienced incarceration. The studies reported on in this chapter control for a variety of socioeconomic characteristics, indicating that parental incarceration, independent of other factors, causes children to do worse cognitively and non-cognitively.[1]

Association of parental incarceration with children's cognitive outcomes

Children with incarcerated parents are 33 per cent more likely to have speech or language problems such as stuttering or stammering than other-wise similar children whose fathers have not been incarcerated (Turney 2014). The grade averages of children also decline after a parent becomes incarcerated (Foster and Hagan 2009). Controlling for race, IQ, home quality, poverty status, and mother's education, it is more common for children of incarcerated parents to drop out of school than it is for children of non-incarcerated parents (Aaron and Dallaire 2010, Nichols and Loper 2012). This is especially true for boys between the ages of 11 and 14 with a mother behind bars. A Chicago-based study indicates that boys are 25 per cent more likely to drop out of school, and they are 55 per cent more likely to drop out of school because they themselves have been incarcerated (Cho 2010). The children of incarcerated fathers complete fewer years of school than children of non-incarcerated fathers, controlling for other likely confounding social and demographic characteristics. The statistical methods used to determine this are sufficiently sophisticated to suggest that the paternal incarceration itself is the cause of children completing fewer years of education than children of never-incarcerated fathers (Foster and Hagan 2009).

Association of parental incarceration with non-cognitive outcomes

Incarceration has also been shown to affect children's non-cognitive outcomes. The children of parents who have been incarcerated are more prone to learning disabilities (defined as a limitation in activities because of a medical, behavioural or other condition) than are children whose parents were never behind bars (Turney 2014). Children with incarcerated parents are 48 per cent more likely to be diagnosed with attention deficit hyperactivity disorder (ADHD) than children with non-incarcerated parents (Turney 2014). They are 23 per cent more likely to suffer from developmental delays (Turney 2014). Children with incarcerated parents, especially the sons of incarcerated fathers, are 43 per cent more likely to suffer from behavioural problems (Johnson 2009, Turney 2014). These differences show up in comparisons of otherwise similar children, even those who experience other disruptive events such as parental divorce or death, and after accounting for other characteristics that are generally understood to cause learning disabilities (Johnson 2009, Turney 2014).

Figure 14.3 summarises findings from studies that describe the increased likelihood that children of parents who have ever been incarcerated will have various negative health, development and education

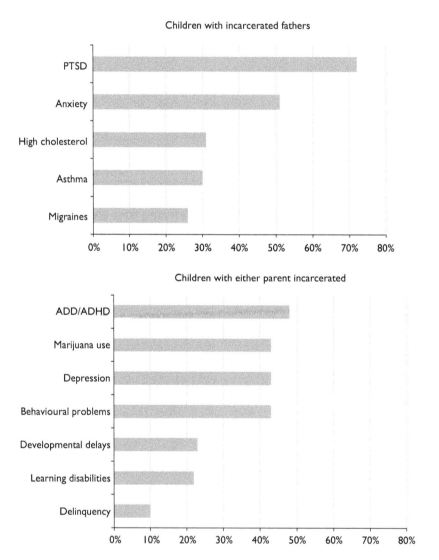

Figure 14.3 The greater likelihood that children with incarcerated parents will experience physical and mental health problems.

outcomes, in comparison with the likelihood that children of never-incarcerated parents will have them (Aaron and Dallaire 2010, Lee *et al.* 2013, Turney 2014, Mears and Siennick 2016).

The children of incarcerated fathers suffer from worse physical health: they are a quarter to a third more likely than children of non-incarcerated fathers to suffer from migraine, asthma and high cholesterol (Lee *et al.* 2013). Their mental health is also worse than that of children of non-incarcerated fathers: the children of incarcerated fathers are 51 per cent more likely to suffer from anxiety, 43 per cent more likely to suffer from depression and 72 per cent more likely to suffer from post-traumatic stress disorder (Lee *et al.* 2013).

As adults, the daughters of parents who have been incarcerated have a higher body mass index, which is associated with other health problems, such as heart disease and diabetes. For example, a 150-pound, 5-foot, 6-inch, 28-year-old woman has a predicted greater weight of 9 pounds if, when she was a child, her parent was incarcerated (Roettger and Board-man 2012). The children of incarcerated parents are also more likely to engage in behaviour that renders them likely to fall victim to the criminal justice system. For example, they are 43 per cent more likely than socially and demographically similar children of non-incarcerated parents to use marijuana (Mears and Siennick 2016). They are 10 per cent more likely to engage in anti-social or delinquent behaviour than children without incarcerated parents (Geller *et al.* 2009, Aaron and Dallaire 2010, Murray, Loeber and Pardini 2012). And finally, children of incarcerated parents are at greater risk of themselves being imprisoned (with the risk of incarceration being greatest for children of incarcerated mothers) (Dallaire 2007, Huebner and Gustafson 2007).

Plausible pathways between parental incarceration and negative outcomes for children

Parental incarceration is independently likely to result in worse outcomes for children for a variety of causes, including socioeconomic factors, psychological and family factors, and health influences.

Socioeconomic pathways

It has been shown that the children of incarcerated parents experience more economic instability and are more likely themselves to become poor (Johnson 2009). Prior to their incarceration, more than half of all inmates were the primary income providers for their families (Western and Pettit 2010). But prisoners make little or no money, so incarceration usually means a sharp decline in (or the complete loss of) family income. Financial distress continues after release from prison because finding a job can be difficult. In the USA, a criminal record can formally and informally bar former prisoners from employment (Western and Pettit 2010, Wright 2013). Formerly imprisoned African-American men without a high school education earn substantially less than African-American men with similarly low educational attainment but without a criminal record (Schanzenbach *et al.* 2016). Parent income is a strong predictor of how children will fare in school and, thus, into adulthood (College Board 2015, Chmielewski and Reardon 2016).

Income losses from incarceration and exclusion from post-incarceration employment can cause multi-generational harm, because upward income mobility – in the form of an individual or a family's improvement in their economic standing – is relatively rare, and it is especially rare for African-Americans. The USA has less intergenerational mobility than many other industrialised societies. Of US children born to parents with incomes in the bottom income quintile, almost half (43 per cent) remain trapped in the bottom quintile as adults and only 30 per cent make it to the middle quintile or higher. African-Americans have even less mobility. For those born to parents in the bottom income quintile, over half (53 per cent) remain there as adults, and only a quarter (26 per cent) make it to the middle quintile or higher (Lopoo and DeLeire 2012). These estimates compare the average income of parents over a five-year period with the average income of their children when these children are approximately the same age as the parents were when the initial income data were collected. In other words, incarceration not only predicts worse outcomes for prisoners' children, but also for their grandchildren and beyond.

Family and psychological pathways

Visiting a parent behind bars is stressful. There is usually no place to play. Waiting times can be long. Sometimes, physical contact between child and parent is limited or prohibited (Murray, Farrington and Sekol 2012). In combination, these are traumatic influences on a child's social, intellectual and emotional development. After a parent is incarcerated, the remaining parent is likely to experience higher stress levels than before their partner was imprisoned (Aaron and Dallaire 2010). When a father is incarcerated, the remaining parent, the mother, may need to work longer hours, making her less available to her child. As a result, the non-incarcerated parent is likely less able to pay attention to their child. Children of incarcerated parents are also likely to be unsupervised more frequently than children of non-incarcerated parents (Aaron and Dallaire 2010).

When a parent becomes incarcerated, family conflict tends to increase (Aaron and Dallaire, 2010). Such conflict and instability in parents' relationships as a result of the incarceration puts children at heightened risk of misbehaving, including at school (Aaron and Dallaire 2010). Because of challenging externalising behaviour, the children of incarcerated parents are more likely to be suspended or even expelled from school, and these consequences frequently deteriorate into delinquency (Johnson 2009, Aaron and Dallaire 2010).

In the context of institutions such as schools and churches, which are meant to be socially supportive, a parent's incarceration is often kept hidden for fear of social stigmatisation (Alexander 2012). The children of incarcerated parents may therefore have fewer opportunities to benefit from resources that are important for social integration. Social relationships and systems are fractured, including both the structures of family and home. Children of incarcerated parents experience greater residential instability, as the remaining parent typically can no longer afford the family's previous housing and must either find a new, less costly, and usually less adequate place for the family to live; move in with relatives; or place children in foster care (Geller *et al.* 2009). Each of these conditions has also been shown to predict children's misbehaviour, suspension and expulsion from school (Johnson 2009).

In the USA, the children of incarcerated mothers are especially likely to end up in foster care (Wildeman 2014). The recent increase in rates of maternal incarceration has added about 100,000 children to the foster care system, close to a third of the increase in the number of fostered children between 1985 and 2000 (Swann and Sylvester 2006, Cho 2010). In general, children in foster care do worse in school than socioeconomically and demographically similar children who are living with a parent (Lesnick *et al.* 2010, Casanueva *et al.* 2012, Barrat and Berliner 2013, Cutuli *et al.* 2013). They are absent from school more frequently and exhibit more behavioural problems (Conger and Rebeck 2001, Harden 2004, Dozier *et al.* 2006, Fisher *et al.* 2006, Casanueva *et al.* 2012).

The children of incarcerated parents, especially incarcerated fathers, are more likely than otherwise similar children to end up homeless, and the homelessness trend is especially pronounced for African-American children of incarcerated fathers (Wildeman 2014). Because they are more likely to move around, live in housing shelters and perhaps sleep on the street, non-incarcerated family members are more likely to be victims of crime (Aaron and Dallaire 2010). Children who are homeless are more likely to do worse in school than otherwise similar children who are not homeless (Fantuzzo *et al.* 2012).

Health pathways

Stress, especially the damaging stress that occurs when a parent is incarcerated, leads to deterioration in mental and physical health, with anxiety, depression and post-traumatic stress disorder being common manifestations (Shonkoff *et al.* 2012). Parental incarceration also provokes or exacerbates family poverty, which itself elevates the stress hormone levels of infants and children (Shonkoff *et al.* 2012). When environmentally challenging conditions, such as the conditions of poverty, chronically elevate stress hormones, the metabolic system can become disrupted, leading to increased risk of dietary disorders including obesity (Burke *et al.* 2011). It has been shown that children who grow up with the chronic stress of poverty often have disrupted brain activity. The principal areas of the brain that are disordered are responsible for emotional regulation, anxiety and memory (Shonkoff *et al.* 2012, Kim *et al.* 2013).

Psychological factors, including a child's own mental and emotional state as well as their mother's, can trigger the onset of asthma as well as worsen the disease (Exley *et al.* 2015). If a mother is emotionally unwell – for example, if she is dealing with the stress of her partner's incarceration – her mental state may increase her child's physiological response to harmful external stimuli as well as disrupt the child's hormonal production (Tibosch *et al.* 2011, Bahreinian *et al.* 2013, Exley *et al.* 2015). The child may appear fine superficially, but these internal biological changes can contribute to the later onset of conditions such as asthma (Wolf *et al.* 2008). Family disruption and diminished resources may mean that children are taken to a doctor less often than is recommended. This, too, may contribute to poor health. The relationships between incarceration and family harm can therefore become cyclical: a parent is incarcerated, the family income drops, housing stability is eroded and stress increases. Children do worse in school and their health deteriorates. They drop out or are expelled. They become delinquent or homeless, or end up in foster care. Eventually, they may find themselves in trouble with the law, and their children may suffer the same consequences as they themselves have faced.

Practical justice interventions: some ways forward

The incarceration of African-Americans in the USA has taken place on such a massive scale that even those policymakers who recognise the problem are paralysed in their consideration of how to address it. The incremental approach that US policymakers usually take to addressing social problems is wholly inadequate to the task of integrating into mainstream society the extraordinary number of African-American men and their families who have been unjustly caught up in the penal system. Progress requires, however, recognition that something is wrong, that careful attention needs to be given to the nature and causes of the problem, and that remedies may be required at several different levels in order to effect change. Together, these elements constitute key elements which might be understood as a practical justice approach.

There are no simple formulae for reducing the incentives for prosecutors of those charged with violent crimes to seek prison terms that are excessive by historical standards and are not needed to deter or prevent crime. In the case of the war on drugs, however, reforms are easier to design and implement (Pfaff 2015). For example, one of the more serious racially discriminatory aspects of the criminal justice system is the difference between the sentences given for crimes involving crack or powder cocaine, two chemically identical substances. African-Americans tend to use crack cocaine, and whites tend to use powder (*Dorsey v United States* 2012, *Hill v United States* 2012). In 1986, the US Congress adopted minimum sentences for possession of crack cocaine that were 100 times more severe than the sentences for possession of powder cocaine: a person arrested with 5 grams of crack cocaine faced a five-year mandatory minimum sentence, while one arrested with powder cocaine did not face the same five-year sentence unless they possessed 500 grams. This obvious racial disparity was upheld by courts because, under current legal doctrines, racial discrimination can be proven only if those enacting the law openly stated that their purpose was to discriminate on the basis of race. In 2010, Congress reduced the disparity from a ratio of 100-to-1 to 18-to-1 and also slightly reduced mandatory minimums. These compromises had no rational basis, and they preserve the severe sentencing and mass incarceration of African-Americans. The ratio should be eliminated entirely (Holder 2016).

A rather different practical justice approach to reducing the effects of parental incarceration on children lies in the elimination of mandatory minimum sentences for non-violent crimes. Especially for those offenders who commit property offences, such as petty theft, alternative forms of correction, can reduce re-offending (Hamilton Project 2014). Enhanced parole, for instance, is a system of prisoner release which includes post-imprisonment support systems such as employment assistance and job training, counselling, substance abuse treatment, parenting classes, family counselling, budgeting classes, housing assistance and help applying for government benefits (Veysey *et al.* 2014). In fact, there is evidence that not incarcerating petty criminals has more social and economic benefits than it has costs (Raphael and Stoll 2014).

When prisoners are released, concrete policies and programmes can alleviate the damages of incarceration on families. Social support and family-based interventions can help prevent family strain and breakdown and foster reunification of families. In the state of Hawaii, for instance, a law calls on the Department of Public Safety to provide parenting classes for inmates, and, attempts are made to keep inmates incarcerated within close geographical proximity to their families (Annie E. Casey Foundation 2016).

To minimise the effects of criminal records on formerly incarcerated people's chance of securing employment, states should require employers to delay questions about applicants' criminal records until after they have settled on preferred job candidates. Such a process, already implemented in over 100 cities and many states, yields an increase in hiring people with criminal records (Annie E. Casey Foundation 2016). When formerly incarcerated parents secure a job, it is more likely that they are able to support their families and attenuate the economic, emotional and social strain as a result of post-incarceration unemployment.

The Children of Incarcerated Parents Bill of Rights was developed with the explicit purpose of incorporating a focus on children in criminal justice reform (San Francisco Children of Incarcerated Parents Partnership n.d.). In fact, strong family bonds upon re-entry into the community can deter further crime (Listwan *et al.* 2006). And yet, there are too few such supports in place (Comfort *et al.* 2016). Reformers have paid too little attention to designing prisoner re-entry programmes that give special attention to the needs of children. One notable programme, however, called Girls Scouts Beyond Bars, provides support to girls with incarcerated mothers, including promoting connections between mother and daughter, planning for a mother's re-entry into the wider community, and connecting the daughters of incarcerated mothers to community services (John *et al.* 2011). Reform should consider the development of more programmes such as these that seek to promote positive family relationships and children's wellbeing.

Conclusion

Children's cognitive and non-cognitive problems, to which parental incarceration contributes, and the concentration of children of incarcerated parents in low-income minority neighbourhoods and in segregated schools, create challenges for teachers and schools that are difficult to overcome. Because of its effects on children, the mass incarceration of African-American men in the USA contributes to the relatively low average performance of African-American children. The practical justice implications of this process of mass incarceration are important and urgent. The social, epidemiological and medical science scholarship this chapter reports on is well positioned to lead us to improve our capacity to address the underlying unjust causes and consequences of excessive imprisonment. When carefully implemented and at scale, research- and practical-justice-based policy and programmatic approaches to the problem of discriminatory incarceration hold the potential to contribute to large-scale social change.

Acknowledgement

An earlier version of this chapter was previously published on the Economic Policy Institute website as Morsy, L., and Rothstein, R., 2016. *Mass Incarceration and Children's Outcomes: Criminal Justice Policy is Education Policy.* Washington, DC: Economic Policy Institute. Elements of this earlier paper are reproduced here with permission.

Note

1 For controls see Aaron and Dallaire (2010, p. 1480), Cho (2010, p. 264), Murray, Loeber and Pardini (2012, p. 282), Roettger and Boardman (2012, p. 639), Lee *et al.* (2013, p. 1192), Lee *et al.* (2014, p. 52), Turney (2014, p. 30), and Mears and Siennick (2016, p. 21).

References

Aaron, L. and Dallaire, D. H., 2010. Parental Incarceration and Multiple Risk Experiences: Effects on Family Dynamics and Children's Delinquency. *Journal of Youth and Adolescence*, 39 (12), 1471–1484.

Alexander, M., 2012. *The New Jim Crow: Mass Incarceration in the Age of Colorblindness.* New York: The New Press.

Amici Curiæ from the American Civil Liberties Union Supporting Petitioners Dorsey and Hill, in *Hill v. United States*, US 11-5721 and *Dorsey v. United States*, US 11-5683 (2012).

Annie E. Casey Foundation, 2016. *A Shared Sentence: The Devastating Toll of Parental Incarceration on Kids, Families, and Communities.* Baltimore, MD: Annie E. Casey Foundation.

Bahreinian, S., Ball, G. D., Vander Leek, T. K., Colman, I., McNeil, B. J., Becker, A. B. and Kozyrskyj, A. L., 2013. Allostatic Load Biomarkers and Asthma in Adolescents. *American Journal of Respiratory and Critical Care Medicine*, 187 (2), 144–152.

Barrat, V. X. and Berliner, B., 2013. *The Invisible Achievement Gap, Part 1: Education Outcomes of Students in Foster Care in California's Public Schools.* San Francisco: WestEd.

Blumstein, A. and Beck, A. J., 1999. Population Growth in U.S. Prisons, 1980–1996. *Crime and Justice*, 26, 17–61.

Bonczar, T. P., 2003. *Prevalence of Imprisonment in the U.S. Population: 1974–2001.* Washington, DC: U.S. Department of Justice.

Burke, N. J., Hellman, J. L., Scott, BG., Weems, C. F. and Carrion, V. G., 2011. The Impact of Adverse Childhood Experiences on an Urban Pediatric Population. *Child Abuse & Neglect*, 35 (6), 408–413.

Carson, E. A., 2015. *Prisoners in 2014.* Washington, DC: U.S. Department of Justice.

Casanueva, C., Wilson, E., Smith, K., Dolan, M., Ringeisen, H. and Horne, B., 2012. *NSCAW II Wave 2 Report: Child Well-being.* (OPRE Report No. 2012-38). Washington, DC: Office of Planning, Research and Evaluation, Administration for Children and Families, U.S. Department of Health and Human Services.

Chmielewski, A. K. and Reardon, S. F., 2016. Patterns of Cross-national Variation in the Association between Income and Academic Achievement. *AERA Open*, 2 (3), doi: 2332858416649593.

Cho, R. M., 2010. Maternal Incarceration and Children's Adolescent Outcomes: Timing and Dosage. *Social Service Review*, 84 (2), 257–282.

College Board, 2015. *Total Group Profile Report: 2015 College-bound Seniors.* New York: The College Board.

Comfort, M., McKay, T., Landwehr, J., Kennedy, E., Lindquist, C. and Bir, A., 2016. *Parenting and Partnership when Fathers Return from Prison: Findings from Qualitative Analysis.* (No. ASPE Research Brief). Washington, DC: Office of the Assistant Secretary for Planning and Evaluation, U.S. Department of Health and Human Services.

Conger, D. and Rebeck, A., 2001. *How Children's Foster Care Experiences Affect Their Education*. New York: Vera Institute of Justice, New York City Administration for Children's Services.

Cutuli, J. J., Desjardins, C. D., Herbers, J. E., Masten, A. S., Long, J. D., Chan, C.-K., Heistad, D. and Hinz, E., 2013. Academic Achievement Trajectories of Homeless and Highly Mobile Students: Resilience in the Context of Chronic and Acute Risk. *Child Development*, 84 (3), 841–857.

Dallaire, D. H., 2007. Incarcerated Mothers and Fathers: A Comparison of Risks for Children and Families. *Family Relations*, 56 (5), 440–453.

Dozier, M., Manni, M. and Gordon, M., 2006. Foster Children's Diurnal Production of Cortisol: An Exploratory Study. *Child Maltreatment*, 11 (2), 189–197.

Exley, D., Norman, A. and Hyland, M., 2015. Adverse Childhood Experience and Asthma Onset: A Systematic Review. *European Respiratory Review*, 24 (136), 299–305.

Fantuzzo, J. W., Le Bœuf, W. A., Chen, C. -C., Rouse, H. L. and Culhane, D. P., 2012. The Unique and Combined Effects of Homelessness and School Mobility on the Educational Outcomes of Young Children. *Educational Researcher*, 41 (9), 393–402.

Fisher, P. A., Gunnar, M. R., Dozier, M., Bruce, J. and Pears, K. C., 2006. Effects of Therapeutic Interventions for Foster Children on Behavioral Problems, Caregiver Attachment, and Stress Regulatory Neural Systems. *Annals of the New York Academy of Sciences*, 1094 (1), 215–225.

Foster, H. and Hagan, J., 2009. The Mass Incarceration of Parents in America: Issues of Race/Ethnicity, Collateral Damage to Children, and Prisoner Reentry. *Annals of the American Academy of Political and Social Science*, 623 (1), 179–194.

Geller, A., Garfinkel, I., Cooper, C. E. and Mincy, R. B., 2009. Parental Incarceration and Child Well-being: Implications for Urban Families. *Social Science Quarterly*, 90 (5), 1186–1202.

Hamilton Project, 2014. A New Approach to Reducing Incarceration While Maintaining Low Rates of Crime. *Policy Brief Series, 2014* (3), 1.

Harden, B. J., 2004. Safety and Stability for Foster Children: A Developmental Perspective. *Future of Children*, 14 (1), 31–47.

Holder, E. H. J., 2016. We Can Have Shorter Sentences and Less Crime. *New York Times*, 14 August. Available from: www.nytimes.com/2016/08/14/opinion/sunday/eric-h-holder-mandatory-minimum-sentences-full-of-errors.html [Accessed 4 June 2018].

Huebner, B. M. and Gustafson, R., 2007. The Effect of Maternal Incarceration on Adult Offspring Involvement in the Criminal Justice System. *Journal of Criminal Justice*, 35 (3), 283–296.

John, D. S. J., Herman, T. S. and Baker, W. L., 2011. *The Effects of Parental Incarceration on Children: Needs and Responsive Services: Report of the Advisory Committee Pursuant to House Resolution 203 and Senate Resolution 52 of 2009*. Harrisburg, PA: General Assembly of the Commonwealth of Pennsylvania.

Johnson, R., 2009. Ever-increasing Levels of Parental Incarceration and the Consequences for Children. In: S. Raphael and M. A. Stoll, eds, *Do Prisons Make Us Safer? The Benefits and Costs of the Prison Boom*. New York: The Russell Sage Foundation, 177–206.

Kim, P., Evans, G. W., Angstadt, M., Ho, S. S., Sripada, C. S., Swain, J. E., Liberson, I. and Luan Phan, K., 2013. Effects of Childhood Poverty and Chronic Stress on Emotion Regulatory Brain Function in Adulthood. *Proceedings of the National Academy of Sciences of the United States of America*, 110 (46), 18442–18447. doi: 10.1073/pnas.1308240110.

Lee, R. D., Fang, X. and Luo, F., 2013. The Impact of Parental Incarceration on the Physical and Mental Health of Young Adults. *Pediatrics*, 131 (4), e1195. doi: 10.1542/peds.2012-0627.

Lesnick, J., George, R. M. Smithgall, C. and Gwynne, J., 2010. *Reading on Grade Level in Third Grade: How Is It Related to High School Performance and College Enrollment*. Chicago: Chapin Hall at the University of Chicago.

Listwan, S. J., Cullen, F. T. and Latessa, E. J., 2006. How to Prevent Prisoner Reentry Programs from Failing: Insights from Evidence-based Corrections. *Federal Probation*, 70 (3), 19–25.

Lopoo, L. and DeLeire, T., 2012. *Pursuing the American Dream: Economic Mobility across Generations*. Washington, DC: The Pew Charitable Trusts.

Makarechi, K., 2015. What the Data Really Says about Police and Racial Bias. *Vanity Fair*, 14 July. Available from: www.vanityfair.com/news/2016/07/data-police-racial-bias [Accessed 4 June 2018].

Mears, D. P. and Siennick, S. E., 2016. Young Adult Outcomes and the Life-course Penalties of Parental Incarceration. *Journal of Research in Crime and Delinquency*, 53 (1), 3–35. doi: 10.1177/0022427815592452.

Murray, J., Farrington, D. P. and Sekol, I., 2012. Children's Antisocial Behavior, Mental Health, Drug Use, and Educational Performance after Parental Incarceration: A Systematic Review and Meta-analysis. *Psychological Bulletin*, 138 (2), 175–210. doi: 10.1037/a0026407.

Murray, J., Loeber, R. and Pardini, D., 2012. Parental Involvement in the Criminal Justice System and the Development of Youth Theft, Marijuana Use, Depression, and Poor Academic Performance. *Criminology*, 50 (1), 255–302.

Nichols, E. B. and Loper, A. B., 2012. Incarceration in the Household: Academic Outcomes of Adolescents with an Incarcerated Household Member. *Journal of Youth and Adolescence*, 41 (11), 1455–1471.

Pfaff, J. F., 2015. The War on Drugs and Prison Growth: Limited Importance, Limited Legislative Options. *Harvard Journal on Legislation*, 52 (1), 173.

Prison Policy Initiative, 2016. *United States Incarceration Rates by Race and Ethnicity, 2010*. Available from: www.prisonpolicy.org/graphs/raceinc.html [Accessed 2 June 2018].

Raphael, S. and Stoll, M. A., 2014. A New Approach to Reducing Incarceration While Maintaining Low Rates of Crime. *Discussion Paper Series*, 2014 (3), 1.

Robles, F. and Dewan, S., 2015. Skip Child Support. Go to Jail. Lose Job. Repeat. *New York Times*, 20 April, A1. Available from: www.nytimes.com/2015/04/20/us/skip-child-support-go-to-jail-lose-job-repeat.html [Accessed 4 June 2018].

Roettger, M. E. and Boardman, J. D., 2012. Parental Incarceration and Gender-based Risks for Increased Body Mass Index: Evidence from the National Longitudinal Study of Adolescent Health in the United States. *American Journal of Epidemiology*, 175 (7), 636–644. doi: 10.1093/aje/kwr409.

San Francisco Children of Incarcerated Parents Partnership, n.d. Available from: www.sfcipp.org/ [Accessed 2 June 2018].

Schanzenbach, D. W., Nunn, R., Bauer, L., Breitwieser, A., Mumford, M., Nantz, G. and the Hamilton Project, 2016. *Twelve Facts about Incarceration and Prisoner Reentry*. Washington, DC: The Hamilton Project, Brookings.

Sentencing Project, 2017. *Trends in U.S. Corrections: U.S. State and Federal Prison Population, 1925–2015*. Washington, DC: The Sentencing Project.

Shonkoff, J. P., Garner, A. S., Siegel, B. S., Dobbins, M. I., Earls, M. F., McGuinn, L., Pascoe, J. and Wood, D. L., 2012. The Lifelong Effects of Early Childhood Adversity and Toxic Stress. *Pediatrics*, 129 (1), 232. doi: 10.1542/peds.2011-2663.

Swann, C. A. and Sylvester, M. S., 2006. The Foster Care Crisis: What Caused Caseloads to Grow. *Demography*, 43 (2), 309–335.

Tibosch, M. M., Verhaak, C. M. and Merkus, P. J., 2011. Psychological Characteristics Associated with the Onset and Course of Asthma in Children and Adolescents: A Systematic Review of Longitudinal Effects. *Patient Education and Counseling*, 82 (1), 11–19.

Turney, K., 2014. Stress Proliferation across Generations? Examining the Relationship between Parental Incarceration and Childhood Health. *Journal of Health and Social Behavior*, 55 (3), 302–319. doi: 10.1177/0022146514544173.

Veysey, B. M., Ostermann, M. and Lanterman, J. L., 2014. The Effectiveness of Enhanced Parole Supervision and Community Services: New Jersey's Serious and Violent Offender Reentry Initiative. *The Prison Journal*, 94 (4), 435–453.

Wagner, P. and Walsh, A., 2016. *States of Incarceration: The Global Context 2016*. Available from: www.prisonpolicy.org/global/2016.html [Accessed 2 June 2018].

Western, B. and Pettit, B., 2010. *Collateral Costs: Incarceration's Effect on Economic Mobility*. Washington, DC: The Pew Charitable Trusts.

Wildeman, C., 2014. Parental Incarceration, Child Homelessness, and the Invisible Consequences of Mass Imprisonment. *Annals of the American Academy of Political and Social Science*, 651 (1), 74–96.

Wildeman, C. and Western, B., 2010. Incarceration in Fragile Families. *Future of Children*, 20 (2), 157–177.

Wolf, J. M., Miller, G. E. and Chen, E., 2008. Parent Psychological States Predict Changes in Inflammatory Markers in Children with Asthma and Healthy Children. *Brain, Behavior, and Immunity*, 22 (4), 433–441.

Wright, K., 2013. Boxed in: How a Criminal Record Keeps You Unemployed for Life. *The Nation*, 25 November. Available from: www.thenation.com/article/boxed-how-criminal-record-keeps-you-unemployed-life/ [Accessed 4 June 2018].

Chapter 15

Antimicrobial resistance, bacterial relations and social justice

Alex Broom, Assa Doron and Peter Aggleton

Introduction

Antimicrobial resistance (AMR) is emerging as the most critical health challenge of the twenty-first century. It is, at one level, a natural evolutionary process. Genes conferring resistance against antibiotics existed long before the use of antibiotic medicines, and have been isolated from glaciers 2,000 years old. But AMR has in recent years been greatly accelerated by human actions and misuse. It is this key concern – the cultural production of AMR and its implications for social justice – that we explore in this chapter.

In order to understand AMR as a cultural problem, it is useful to begin with the socio-historical context to its emergence. The global challenge of resistance, currently being emphasised by pan-national and peak national organisations, including the World Health Organization[1] (WHO), the European Union[2] (EU) and the US Centers for Disease Control and Prevention[3] (US CDC), was anticipated by scientists even in the early years of antimicrobials. In fact, the threat of resistance outlined in Alexander Fleming's Nobel Prize speech for the discovery of penicillin on 11 December 1945 was prescient when he declared:

> It is not difficult to make microbes resistant to penicillin in the laboratory by exposing them to concentrations not sufficient to kill them ... There is the danger that the ignorant man may easily underdose himself and by exposing his microbes to non-lethal quantities of the drug, make them resistant.[4]

While Fleming in this account focused on only one dimension of the problem – under-dosing – his concerns around inappropriate use were warranted. Fleming was acutely aware of the potential for his discovery to have diminishing potency: as was Andrew Moyer, who perfected a method for its mass production in the USA; Howard Florey, the Australian pharmacologist, who developed a powdery form of penicillin; and Ernst Chain, the German-born British biochemist, who assisted Florey (Hall *et al.* 2018). Fleming's prediction was of course correct: bacteria – and some more than others – had an uncanny ability to evolve in relation to antimicrobials over time. Consider, for instance, the fact that penicillin-resistant staphylococcal infection was first detected in 1940, while still being given to relatively few patients. Tetracycline was introduced in 1950, and tetracycline-resistant Shigella, which causes a form of dysentery, materialised in 1959. Erythromycin came on the market in 1953, and erythromycin-resistant streptococcal infection appeared in 1968. And so the story continues, while fewer classes of antimicrobials were discovered over time. Moreover, as antibiotics became more affordable in many countries and communities (including in farming and lifestock), their use has increased, and thus selective pressure accelerated the further development of AMR.

The discovery and investment in the development of antibiotics received a boost in the Second World War, with large-scale collaboration of government and industry in the mass production for use in conflict zones in particular. The post-war period then saw a 'golden age of antibiotics' (Hall *et al.* 2018, p. 24), with huge penicillin-producing factories built in the USA, a thriving pharmaceutical industry, and little consideration of cost over time (or diminishing returns resulting from selective pressure and resistance). Antibiotics were celebrated for reducing the fatalities of war and as presenting a miracle cure for previously intractable infectious diseases. This golden age ensured that any concerns around antibiotic resistance were little more than 'background noise' – hardly considered by politicians, industry or even physicians, let alone the laypersons.

The beginnings of a global response

In 2015, the WHO announced a Global Action Plan, and the director general warned of the dire consequences of AMR. In 2017, the UN General Assembly met specifically to discuss the threat of AMR. According to the United States Centres for Disease Control report (Centres for Disease Control and Prevention 2013) there were approximately 23,000 deaths in the USA alone from resistant organisms each year (and increasing), with a highly controversial report published by KPMG[5] projecting that by 2050 antimicrobial-resistant infections may contribute to as many as 10 million deaths per year. What, then, are the solutions currently proposed?

The response of the WHO as well as most other key international stakeholders has been to emphasise the need to urgently solve the following two problems: (1) the ongoing inappropriate use of medicines; and (2) the stagnating pipeline for new antibiotics. These issues are of course enmeshed – without improving use, any pharmaceuticals developed will quickly have diminishing returns. Thus, while we know that in tackling AMR, technical and biological solutions are required, there is also widespread acceptance that the problem of resistance is now largely driven by human activities, creating selective pressure – a process which enables resistant strains to thrive and spread easily. This makes AMR a social, cultural, economic and political concern as much as a biological or medical puzzle. However, in seeking to redress the threat of AMR, as we will posit in this chapter, we must also contend with questions of social justice; and specifically how the threat of AMR disproportionally affects low-income countries or, in turn, how action requires *disproportionate responsiveness* from economically poorer countries.

While the social dimensions of antimicrobial resistance are gaining interest in the social sciences (e.g. Broom *et al.* 2014, 2015, 2017, 2018), rather less attention has been paid to the intersection of the global threat posed by AMR, the rise of 'optimisation' tactics (e.g. governance, surveillance or restriction of antimicrobials) as a strategy for ameliorating resistance, and the everyday practices of use as embedded in the contextual specificities of low- and middle-income countries. This includes, importantly, how any global response must be shaped by understandings of local constraints, vulnerabilities and fairness/justice, and, moreover, how the story of antibiotics – their rise and impending fall – mirrors the broader relationship between the global North and South. Specifically, the cultural history of antibiotics (and their decline) is in many respects a story of their (over)consumption and overuse in OECD countries, rather than a problem of current-day misuse in economically poorer countries. In practice, this means that what is often being asked of many economically poorer countries (i.e. to tighten governance, restrict access and use), in the context of current demands for judicious and rational use, sits in stark contrast to the practices of the First World throughout much of the twentieth and twenty-first centuries. Justice in this context lies in the geopolitical (global) demands for change, and the extent to which considerations of 'comparative' advantage, responsibility, histories of (mis)use and capacity for leadership/improvement must be taken into account.

Perfect policies and harsh realities – the case of India

2012 was a time of considerable political significance for AMR in the Indian context. There was increasing concern about the ramifications of the rise of AMR (and global policies emphasising misuse) in India, a country that was at the time the highest consumer of antibiotics globally. Moreover, purchases of antibiotics were increasing significantly. Recent IQVIA Consulting and Information Services India (formerly IMS Health Information & Consulting Services India) data, for example, suggests that antiobiotic purchases from retail outlets in India rose from 3,763 crore rupees (INR) in 2005 to 5,886 crore rupees (INR) in 2008, and 6,414 crore rupees (INR) in 2009 (Ganguly *et al.* 2011, p. v), and these are only those documented in the formal health sector as compared with the thriving black market for pharmaceuticals.

The Chennai Declaration – the product of a joint meeting of key medical and scientific stakeholders in India (see http://chennaideclaration.org/) – was published in 2013 as an agenda to begin to address AMR in the Indian context. The initial joint meeting in 2012, which led to the Declaration, brought together the Indian National Accreditation Board of Hospitals, the Medical Council of India, the Drug Controller General of India, the Indian Council of Medical Research and the WHO (among others) to discuss the considerable ramifications of AMR for India. This meeting and the Declaration sought to outline a strategy to begin to deal with the problem of resistance and antimiocrobial misuse in the Indian context (and potentially in other developing countries). The Declaration also acknowledged the limits of what could be expected to change in the context of development and structural constraints. The roadmap offered a sober assessment and focused on realistic goals and expectations, asserting, among many other things, that:

> a strict and perfect antibiotic policy is always the ideal, just like having a perfect police and law and order system … asking for a complete and strict antibiotic policy in a country where there is currently no functioning antibiotic policy at all may not be an intelligent or immediately viable option without the political will to make such a drastic change.

This statement captures some of the dimensions of the AMR problem (and its possible solutions) within economically poorer contexts. For example, what can be realistically achieved in relation to the threat of AMR, and in tightening antimicrobial misuse, in the context of existing and entrenched structural problems, and moreover, against the background of weak governance and limited healthcare provision by the state? There was an acute awareness of such limitations in Chennai, and an intention that expectations should be suited to existing broader problems of governance and regulation.

Confronting the issue was ultimately articulated as daunting, both at the policy and the grassroots level. How could India – with hugely varying standards of infection control even in healthcare facilities, a paucity of published data on the existence of antibiotic controls and inaccurate compliance reporting, possibly gain control over the problem of AMR? Even in relatively well-off countries such as the USA and Australia, systematic surveillance of antimicrobials was relatively limited and control poor. For example, at that same time (circa 2012), Australia had no national reporting procedures for multi-resistant organisms in place nor compulsory antimicrobial stewardship (AMS) across all the health sector.

The practical challenges to initiating a pan-Indian response were formidable. As Ghafur and colleagues noted at the time of the Declaration, the country comprised 'more than 20,000 hospitals, more than a billion population, wide cultural diversity, socio-economic disparity, and a large medical community of more than three-fourths of a million doctors' (2012, p. 72). Addressing the misuse of antibiotics in this context was an issue few dared engage with – a situation made evident when an earlier policy developed in 2011 was sidelined because none of the recommendations were viewed as implementable in the Indian context (Ghafur *et al.* 2012, p. 72).

Another twist in the story of AMR in India came in 2009 with the naming of a new 'superbug' called New Delhi metallo-beta-lactamase 1 (NDM-1). First identified in a Swedish tourist who had visited India, its identification and naming was met with anger in the sub-continent, given ambiguity about whether it was in fact of Indian origin. But these events exemplify emergent dynamics in the global response: in the form of the construction of 'villains', 'misusers' and 'successes' in the race to address AMR. This has the potential to position economically poorer countries in a rather dim light, with little consideration of opportunity, context, vulnerability and capacity to enact change.

Below we outline some of the specific structural considerations and cultural practices which help to contextualise the problem of AMR in India (and potentially beyond), but also which highlight the importance of socially just approaches to (global) solutions to AMR. This has practical implications. In the words of the Chennai Declaration, 'India needs an implementable antibiotic policy and NOT a perfect policy' (Ghafur *et al.* 2012, p. 73). Additionally, we posit, any global approach requires a context-sensitive policy, and one that takes into account local constraints.

Low-income populations, access to care and precarious work

Before examining the role of the global pharmaceutical industry in contributing to the rise of AMR in India, it is worth considering broader issues of social inequality. At a fundamental level, the problem of AMR, and in particular the misuse of antimicrobials, is a problem of services, access and vulnerability: factors which intersect both with entrenched dynamics of disadvantage and individual biographies (Kapadia 1995). There is a shortage of well over 500,000 doctors in India, and the ratio of doctors to patients remains well over the 1/1,000 WHO limit (Deo 2013). In contexts of access restriction, it is well documented that it is the poor, marginalised and most vulnerable who are least likely to receive medical care (Baru *et al.* 2010). Likewise, the rise of an Indian middle class (Varma 2007) with increasing demands for higher living standards and a growing capacity to purchase medications, sits at odds with the lack of facilities to provide advice, testing and feedback about optimal antibiotic use.

Layered across this complex landscape are the poor of India whose livelihoods are precarious and access to basic goods haphazard at best (Roy 2005). Over-the-counter, affordable generic medications can be viewed as 'great levellers', especially for poor people, many of whom will resort to antibiotics simply because if they forego a day's work, they are unlikely to find another job (Maiti 2013). Such grassroots realities of infection self-care and prevention amongst the poor touches on the intimate connections between labour, misuse and disadvantage. While global newspaper headlines emphasise that over-the-counter, non-prescription sales of 'last-resort' antibiotics such as the carbapenems in India are a major contributor to growing resistance among Gram-negative organisms globally (see Laxminarayan and Chaudhury 2016), few report the link between antibiotic misuse and everyday survival through precarious forms of work. India's significant rise in consumption of last-resort antimicrobials over the last ten years is thus not merely a governance issue, but a development and social security concern as well.

Herein lies the paradox of AMR we wish to point to: antibiotics can shield an individual temporarily from infection risk in toxic environments and risky labour, but the long-term effects of misuse on the individual and collective can be equally insidious, constituting a form of 'slow violence' (Nixon 2011) that creeps into communities and populations in devastating ways that may be hard to identify and predict. But there is another paradox here when it comes to the relationship between threat and use. That is, the greater the infective threat – and remembering that there are an estimated 58,000 neonatal deaths per year from resistant infections in India (Laxminarayan *et al.* 2016) – the greater the tendency to use antimicrobials. This cycle – driven by the absence of testing for infections, sound advice, knowledge and job security – lies at the core of the AMR problem in the sub-continent.

Toxic environments, infective risks, polluted bodies and AMR

An additional layer of complexity of AMR in India derives from the intersection between environmental pollution and environmental risk. The late twentieth century witnessed the rapid growth of the pharmaceutical industry, with transnational companies migrating factories and production lines to India attracted by regulations and labour conditions favourable to industry. As the result of loose regulatory regimes, pharmaceutical factories routinely discharged effluents replete with antibiotic agents with impunity, contaminating water bodies and the environment. Testing now reveals an unprecedented antimicrobial load within many urban and non-urban environments in India, which feeds the proliferation of multi-resistance organisms (Laxminarayan and Chaudhury 2016, Lübbert *et al.* 2017). This is compounded by extremely high antibiotic use for non-therapeutic purposes in the livestock and agricultural sectors (Kakkar *et al.* 2017). There is therefore a free-for-all market for both legal and illicit antimicrobials in India (Mukherjee 2017). Add this to the aforementioned (and well-known) challenges that Indian populations face, in terms of involvement in risky work and exposure to toxic environments (Doron and Jeffrey 2018), and we can see a 'perfect storm' of infective risk, widespread availability and loose governance.

Securing this as a critical social justice issue, environmental toxicities interplay with other 'toxic environments' in India, including those of slum communities, which have little access to clean water and sanitation. Slum dwellers' participation in 'risky labour' – including India's informal markets of waste-pickers and handlers – involves terrifying working and living conditions, with routine exposure to a variety of infectious agents: a reality poignantly captured by Katherine Boo in her critically acclaimed book, *Behind the Beautiful Forevers* (2014), about a slum community in Mumbai. Other (poorer) Indians participate in highly risky and infection-prone occupations (e.g. sanitation work) and these populations have the least access to formalised medical advice and assistance. Thus, there is a persistent heightened infective risk combined with the inability to access help and care, and with little or no access to basic sanitation facilities. It is not surprising therefore that those who forage on garbage dumps and clean latrines – often known as scavengers – have a very low life expectancy, commonly suffering from respiratory illness and tuberculosis, gastrointestinal disorders and skin infections (Doron and Jeffrey 2018). AMR is likely to dramatically increase risk and mortality for these communities. Under such conditions, it is equally unsurprising that antibiotics assume a 'magical' curative power in lieu of proper diagnosis, with little understanding of the type and dosage required (cf. Chandler *et al.* 2016). It is here that the social justice aspects of addressing the problem of AMR become particularly acute.

In short, the polluted environments of India reflect both the enduring risks of life in the subcontinent, perpetuating established structures of inequality, where lower-caste communities, poor landless labourers and other marginalised communities toil and live under terrible conditions. Concurrently, the toxic landscape reflects India's pull into the global limelight, as the country seeks to capitalise on its 'comparative advantage' to attract foreign investment and become a 'production house' for global pharmaceuticals (and thus their waste, including antibiotics). The global appetite of the rising middle class also makes its demands on the consumer patterns

and increased (and unregulated) use of antibiotics for non-therapeutic purposes to increase food production. This is a major international concern,
especially with recent revelations that colistin – a powerful last-resort antibiotic – is used in poultry farming (Davies and Walsh 2018).

Put all this together, and there is a catostrophic global event in the
making with potentially devastating effects. Many facets of the (urban)
Indian environment (e.g. waterways, sewage outlets) feature much higher
levels of antimicrobials than other contexts (Skariyachan *et al.* 2015),
which contributes to selective pressure for the development of AMR. Completing the cycle of inequality, those most at risk and exposed to polluting
environments (and who are sometimes viewed culturally as 'polluted
citizens') are among the most vulnerable when it comes to efforts to
reduce the availability of non-prescribed antibiotics. Yet, bacteria 'travel',
as recent studies have also shown (e.g. De Lappe *et al.* 2015), and it is
increasingly clear that the spread of multi-resistance organisms exceeds
national boundaries, rendering AMR a politically explosive issue globally,
with implications for migration policy, race relations and border security
(de Smalen *et al.* 2017), as well as profound implications for our collective
capacity to obtain a collectively secure antimicrobial future.

Self-care, privatised healthcare and out-of-pocket expenditure

Despite the intended goals of universal healthcare provision in India
(Patel *et al.* 2015), government funding for healthcare, including treatment for common infections, remains insubstantial and inequitable
(Horton and Das 2011). Out-of-pocket costs for healthcare have increased
over time in both rural and urban areas, resulting in India having one of
the highest proportions worldwide of out-of-pocket expenses for healthcare incurred by individuals (Balarajan *et al.* 2011). The national platform
of limited state healthcare and considerable out-of-pocket expenditure
raises the profile of the intersections of self-care practice in India, vis-à-vis
the global governance agenda. Placing a culture of self-medication alongside an environment of precarious employment (for some) and lack of
formalised healthcare support and care (for many), means that in the
everyday struggle for survival, pragmatism and self-directed pharmaceutical care thrives (augmented by the advice provided by a spectrum of
'streetside' vendors). Herein lie the informal economy and self-care
dimensions of the AMR crisis in India and beyond. Personal expenditure
on healthcare – primarily on pharmaceuticals, including antibiotics (Alsan
et al. 2015) – means that a significant responsibility is placed on the individual in relation to the potential risk of getting an infection (Balarajan *et
al.* 2011, see also Reddy *et al.* 2011). Solutions to AMR thus raise questions
of agency, constraint, structural possibilities and local vulnerabilities.

As indicated earlier, major economic shifts in recent decades have resulted in a growing middle class (Rajan *et al.* 2013) and, in turn, an expansion of private health services, particularly in urban areas (Patel *et al.* 2015). Consumerism is growing in India, which is also evident in the healthcare sector, with 'power' to choose providers placed in the hands of the payee, and to some extent (given this dynamic), the timing and use of antibiotics (and many other interventions).Yet, India continues to display stark inequalities of wealth across place and population (Horton and Das 2011) with considerable variation in access to the private health sector (Shiva *et al.* 2011). Thus this emergent consumerism in India is varied in its manifestations across locale and community. Regardless, the privatisation of healthcare raises questions about the potency (or lack thereof) of the state to enact change in current medication practices and sales (as per the concerns within the Chennai Declaration). However, in turn, there is also variability in the capacity to take action (i.e. differential capacity to purchase pharmaceuticals across gender, caste, education, socioeconomic position, and geographical location) (Broom *et al.* 2009, Balarajan *et al.* 2011). This raises important questions. For example, to what extent is concern around AMR and/or restrained use of antimicrobials realistic in the context of considerable privatisation of healthcare, poor regulation of costs and quality, and unequal economic growth (Patel *et al.* 2015)? Moreover, in contexts where successes in improving healthcare at a population level are skewed largely in favour of the burgeoning middle classes (and the 'urban elite'), where does this leave the poorer populations when faced with the tightening in availability of pharmaceuticals (combined with a rise in resistance within the community – particularly those in risky occupations)?

Discussion

Evident in the global struggle against multi-resistance organisms is a marked insensitivity to socio-economic constraint and population vulnerability. As a result, efforts to tackle multi-resistant organisms globally risk making two key errors: namely, over-emphasising the 'problems' of the developing world (including India), and under-emphasising the drivers of AMR (both in historical and contemporary contexts) in economically wealthier nations. This tendency is highlighted by Hall and colleagues in their recent book, *Superbugs: An Arms Race against Bacteria* (2018), in which they note that of the 40 million people who are given antibiotics for respiratory problems in the USA every year, around 27 million do not need them (p. 3). Such empirical realities provide an important backdrop against which to understand the apparent 'failings' of nations such as India (e.g. Pulla 2017). While it may be tempting for OECD countries to delegate responsibility elsewhere, doing so is both ahistorical (i.e. by ignoring their own use and abuse of antimicrobials, past and present) and places responsibility for change on those who are least able to bring it about.

In contrast to such an approach, greater concern for social justice should underpin efforts to develop solutions to AMR. Using India as a case study, addressing AMR is likely to require a more sophisticated response informed by a commitment to human rights and justice, alongside the political will to avoid further polarisation between the global North and South. If such an approach is not utilised, existing inequalities will likely be further exacerbated by the AMR crisis, with economically poorer countries continuing to be positioned as the unruly 'source of the crisis' and an impediment to change. While the current antibiotic use optimisation agenda in OECD countries espoused by the WHO, EU and the US CDC is largely concerned with tightening control over the availability of antimicrobials and ensuring that they are used appropriately, the case of India provides an important reminder about how context can secure the futility of (simplistic and acontextual) policy interventions. From the perspective of global political economy, the entanglement we can see emerging here can be viewed as anchored in a 'world system' dynamic as Wallerstein and others have argued, whereby the periphery (i.e. developing economies) must carry the burdens of a global political economy steered by core (i.e. rich) nations and their satellites (cf. Wallerstein 1974). Pursuing such an approach evades justice and fairness and will ultimately fail to address this key health challenge of the twenty-first century.

What is needed instead is an approach that brings together broad-ranging and community-specific data concerning the (social and biophyiscal) manifestations of antibiotic resistance and its effects with considered attention to what *should* be done in the context of global inequality if all are to benefit from the actions taken. While we cannot spell out in detail what such an approach might entail in particular countries or regions, a number of elements suggest themselves if we are to pursue a course towards this more practical and equitable form of response. Crucially, our starting point should lie in evidence concerning the inordinate infective risks, environmental exposure and burden of disease (in relation to resistance) amongst (economically) poorer communities and nations. And moreover, how current labour relations, forms of environmental pollution, industrial production and enduring social practices and cultural norms are complicit in the challenge of infective risks and the burden of resistance. Without this knowledge base, little action can be taken to ensure the response to the threat of resistance is sensitive to issues of social justice. Beyond this, however, it will be necessary to consider the costs and benefits of broader health system development – that AMR is not 'solvable' as a problem, without considering the health system (and community) as a whole.

Notes

1 www.who.int/foodsafety/areas_work/antimicrobial-resistance/tripartite/en/.
2 https://ec.europa.eu/health/amr/action_eu_en.
3 www.cdc.gov/onehealth/index.html.
4 www.nobelprize.org/nobel_prizes/medicine/laureates/1945/fleming-lecture. pdf p. 93.
5 https://home.kpmg.com/content/dam/kpmg/pdf/2014/12/amr-report-final. pdf.

References

Alsan, M., Schowmaker, L., Eggleston, K., Kammili, N., Kolli, P. and Bhattacharya, J., 2015. Out-of-Pocket Health Expenditures and Antimicrobial Resistance in Low-income and Middle-income Countries: An Economic Analysis. *Lancet Infectious Diseases*, 15 (10), 1203–1210.

Balarajan, Y., Selvaraj, S. and Subramanian, S. V., 2011. Health Care and Equity in India. *The Lancet*, 377 (9764), 505–515.

Baru, R., Acharya, A., Acharya, S., Shiva Kumar, A. K. and Nagaraj, K., 2010. Inequities in Access to Health Services in India: Caste, Class and Region. *Economic and Political Weekly*, 45 (38), 49–58.

Boo, K., 2014. *Behind the Beautiful Forevers: Life, Death, and Hope in a Mumbai Undercity*. New York: Random House Trade Paperbacks.

Broom, A., Broom, J. and Kirby, E., 2014. Cultures of Resistance? A Bourdieusian Analysis of Doctors' Antibiotic Prescribing. *Social Science and Medicine*, 110, 81–88. doi: 10.1016/j.socscimed.2014.03.030.

Broom, A., Broom, J., Kirby, E. and Scambler, G., 2015. The Path of Least Resistance? Jurisdictions, Responsibility and Professional Asymmetries in Pharmacists' Accounts of Antibiotic Decisions in Hospitals. *Social Science and Medicine*, 146, 95–103. doi: 10.1016/j.socscimed.2015.10.037.

Broom, A., Doron, A. and Tovey, P., 2009. The Inequalities of Medical Pluralism: Hierarchies of Health, the Politics of Tradition and the Economies of Care in Indian Oncology. *Social Science and Medicine*, 69 (5), 698–706.

Broom, A., Kirby, E., Gibson, A., Davis, M. and Broom, J., 2018. The Private Life of Medicine: Accounting for Antibiotics in the 'For-profit' Hospital Setting. *Social Theory and Health*. doi: 10.1057/s41285-018-0063-8.

Broom, A., Kirby, E., Gibson, A., Post, J. J. and Broom, J., 2017. Myth, Manners, and Medical Ritual: Defensive Medicine and the Fetish of Antibiotics. *Qualitative Health Research*, 27 (13), 1994–2005.

Centres for Disease Control and Prevention (US), 2013. *Antibiotic Resistance Threats in the United States, 2013*. Atlanta: Centres for Disease Control and Prevention, US Department of Health and Human Services.

Chandler, C., Hutchinson, E. and Hutchison, C., 2016. *Addressing Antimicrobial Resistance through Social Theory: An Anthropologically Oriented Report*. London: London School of Hygiene and Tropical Medicine. Available from: http://researchonline.lshtm.ac.uk/id/eprint/3400500 [Accessed 6 June 2018].

Davies, M. and Walsh, T., 2018. A Colistin Crisis in India. *The Lancet Infectious Diseases*, 18 (3), 256–257.

De Lappe, N., O'Connor, J., Garvey, P., McKeown, P. and Cormican, M., 2015. Ciprofloxacin-resistant *Shigella sonnei* Associated with Travel to India. *Emerging Infectious Diseases*, 21 (5), 894–896.

Deo, M. G., 2013. Doctor Population Ratio for India: The Reality. *Indian Journal of Medical Research*, 137 (4), 632–635.

Doron, A. and Jeffrey, R., 2018. *Waste of a Nation: Garbage and Growth in India.* Cambridge, MA: Harvard University Press.

Ganguly, N. K. *et al.*, 2011. *Situation Analysis: Antibiotic Use and Resistance in India.* New Delhi: Global Antibiotic Resistance Partnership.

Ghafur, A., Methai, D., Muruganathan, A., Jayalal, J. A., Kant, R., Chaudhary, D., Prabhash, K., Abraham, O. C., Gopalakrishnan, R., Ramasubramanian, V., Shah, S. N., Pardeshi, R., Huilgol, A., Kapil, A., Gill, J., Singh, S., Rissma, H. S., Todi, S., Hegde, B. M. and Parikh, P., 2012. The Chennai Declaration: A Roadmap to Tackle the Challenge of Antimicrobial Resistance. *Indian Journal of Cancer*, 49 (4), 71–81.

Hall, W., McDonnell, A. and O'Neill, J., 2018. *Superbugs: An Arms Race against Bacteria.* Cambridge, MA: Harvard University Press.

Horton, R. and Das, P., 2011. Indian Health: The Path from Crisis to Progress. *The Lancet*, 377 (9761), 181–183.

Kakkar, M., Walia, K., Vong, S., Chatterjee, P. and Sharma, A., 2017. Antibiotic Resistance and Its Containment in India. *British Medical Journal*, 358 (Suppl 1), 25–30.

Kapadia, K., 1995. *Siva and Her Sisters: Gender, Caste, and Class in Rural South India.* Boulder, CO: Westview Press.

Laxminarayan, R. and Chaudhury, R. R., 2016. Antibiotic Resistance in India: Drivers and Opportunities for Action. *PLoS Medicine*, 13 (3), e1001974.

Laxminarayan, R., Matsoso, P., Pant, S., Brower, C., Rottingen, J. -A., Klugman, K. and Davies, S., 2016. Access to Effective Antimicrobials: A Worldwide Challenge. *The Lancet*, 387 (10014), 168–175.

Lübbert, C., Baars, C., Dayakar, A., Lippmann, N., Rodloff, A. C., Kinzig, M. and Sörgel, F., 2017. Environmental Pollution with Antimicrobial Agents from Bulk Drug Manufacturing Industries in Hyderabad, South India. *Infection*, 45 (4), 479–491.

Maiti, D., 2013. Precarious Work in India: Trends and Emerging Issues. *American Behavioral Scientist*, 57 (4), 507–530.

Mukherjee, N., 2017. India Continues to Export Substandard Drugs; Lack of Regulations Real Problem: WHO. *Down to Earth*. Available from: www.downtoearth.org.in/news/substandard-drugs-finding-way-into-global-market-low-income-countries-most-affected-who-59253 [Accessed 6 June 2018].

Nixon, R., 2011. *Slow Violence and the Environmentalism of the Poor.* Cambridge, MA: Harvard University Press.

Patel, V., Parikh, R., Nandraj, S., Balasubramaniam, P., Narayan, K., Paul, V. K., Kumar, A. K., Chatterjee, M. and Reddy, K. S., 2015. Assuring Health Coverage for All in India. *The Lancet*, 386 (10011), 2422–2435.

Pulla, P., 2017. The Superbugs of Hyderabad. *The Hindu*. Available from: www.thehindu.com/opinion/op-ed/the-superbugs-of-hyderabad/article20536685.ece [Accessed 6 June 2018].

Rajan, K., Kennedy, J. and King, L., 2013. Is Wealthier Always Healthier in Poor Countries? The Health Implications of Income, Inequality, Poverty, and Literacy in India. *Social Science and Medicine*, 88, 98–107.

Reddy, K. S., Patel. V., Jha, P., Paul, V. K., Kumar, A. K. and Dandona, L., 2011. Towards Achievement of Universal Health Care in India by 2020: A Call to Action. *The Lancet*, 377 (9767), 760–768.

Roy, T., 2005. *Rethinking Economic Change in India: Labour and Livelihood*. London: Routledge.

Shiva Kumar, A. K., Chen, L. C., Choudhury, M., Ganju, S., Mahajan, V., Sinha, A. and Sen, A., 2011. Financing Health Care for All: Challenges and Opportunities. *The Lancet*, 377 (9766), 668–679.

Skariyachan, S., Mahajanakatti, A. B., Grandhi, N. J., Prasanna, A., Sen, B., Sharma, N., Vasist, K. S. and Narayanappa, R., 2015. Environmental Monitoring of Bacterial Contamination and Antibiotic Resistance Patterns of the Fecal Coliforms Isolated from Cauvery River, a Major Drinking Water Source in Karnataka, India. *Environmental Monitoring and Assessment*, 187 (5), 279.

Smalen de, A. W., Ghorab, H., El Ghany, M. A. and Hill-Cawthorne, G. A., 2017. Refugees and Antimicrobial Resistance: A Systematic Review. *Travel Medicine and Infectious Disease*, 15, 23–28.

Varma, P. K., 2007. *The Great Indian Middle Class*. New Delhi: Penguin Books India.

Wallerstein, I., 1974. *The Modern World System*. New York: The Academic Press.

Chapter 16

Fostering change through the pursuit of practical justice in sexual and reproductive health and rights

Purnima Mane and Peter Aggleton

Introduction

Sexual and reproductive health and rights (SRHR) is a complex and diffi-cult field in which to work, since the issues engaged with arouse strong feelings among politicians, religious leaders, communities and the public alike. All over the world, there are those who adopt a narrow view when it comes to issues such as sex, sexuality, sex relationships – seeing these as private or family matters. But there are others who believe that gender and sexual relations, the prevention and treatment of sexually transmitted infections, and access to contraception and safe abortion are matters of public concern. Over the past 30 years, the HIV epidemic and broader struggles for SRHR have brought many of these matters to the fore, causing governments and communities to confront the fact that gender and sexual inequality and diversity exist, and that without an honest and open approach, little can be achieved. But how should one go about this work in an equitable and honest way, and what can be learned from the successful approaches that have been used to date?

This chapter reflects on some of the changes witnessed over the last few decades in the field of sexual and reproductive health and rights, which provide evidence of how divergent factors can come together to bring about change in an area which has always been characterised by contro-versy and polarisation. Agreeing on a universal definition of sexual and reproductive health and rights (SRHR) has always been difficult (see Chapter 7), and operationalising these rights has been even more complex (see, for instance, Oronje *et al.* 2011).

The current environment is particularly discouraging for many working in this field: we write at a moment when in the USA, access to abortion is increasingly restrictive through additional conditions imposed by different states, such as long waiting periods, multiple visits to the provider, having an ultrasound before the procedure, and minors needing parental permis-sion (Guttmacher Institute 2017). These restrictions extend beyond federal controls and those included in health insurance plans. For instance, just three US states – California, New York and Oregon – mandate that private insurers must cover abortion, with ten states restricting coverage in all private health care plans which are regulated by the state government and 35 states declining to extend state Medicaid funds to cover abortion other than under a few conditions (Donovan 2017).

In respect of a different but no less important set of SRHR concerns, in countries as diverse as Uganda, the Russian Federation and Indonesia, state-sponsored efforts are under way to undermine progress towards the sexual rights of gender and sexual minorities, including same-sex attracted women and men, trans persons and others (Carroll and Mendos 2017). These have had damaging consequences for the individuals concerned, their families and friends and the wider community, turning back progress towards recognition, inclusion and rights, and making it harder for LGBTIQ populations to be reached through health, education and community development programmes and activities.

In struggles for inclusion, respect and justice, it is important to remember the progress and change which has happened in the past – often in extremely difficult conditions and contexts. This chapter is an attempt to do so using two examples – change in the political and social climate to engender a positive response to the HIV epidemic in India, and change in terms of policy reform to ensure that the SRHR of women would be strengthened in Mozambique through access to safe abortion. Analysing these examples through the lens provided by practical justice – with its commitment to the use of scientific evidence, good normative argument and attention to the best vehicles for achieving momentum – can help identify some common factors that foster change even in areas where social and political climates and centuries of embedded prejudice impose formidable barriers.

Early response to the HIV epidemic in India

Informed by rights, evidence, pragmatism and innovation

When AIDS was first identified in India, the initial reaction was a familiar one – namely, that HIV would be a passing epidemic, restricted to certain marginalised populations, then identified as 'risk groups' which had never been the priority of the government. Evidence of prevalence initially was restricted to surveillance sites in red-light districts mainly among sex workers and to a lesser extent among their clients. In the 1980s, limited data existed about sexual health and behaviour, despite an aggressively promoted family planning programme since India's independence 50 years earlier. The fact that health itself and sexual health in particular had received limited attention and resources made the evidence base on sexual health and HIV weaker. The world might well see India as the land of the

Kamasutra and a context in which *hijra* as the 'third sex' have traditionally been assigned a role during the celebration of significant life events. But strong taboos about sex and sexuality co-existed with these practices, making sex and sexuality complex matters for even researchers to address, and adding to the difficulty of not knowing enough about people's sexual behaviour, beliefs and knowledge so as to design effective policies and programmes to address HIV. It did not help that at the time the HIV epidemic was seen as a gay epidemic from the developed world or an 'African problem', with Indian culture(s) of religion and the family believed to have the potential to keep the epidemic at bay.

The multilateral and bilateral donors which funded India's global health and development programmes extensively in the 1980s and early 1990s, however, projected a far worse scenario for India (e.g. World Bank 1993). With a population second only to China and with a range of developmental challenges including high levels of poverty and inequity, low literacy, marked gender inequality and rampant discrimination against populations such as drug users, sex workers and men who have sex with men, health experts and global development agencies were deeply concerned (Mane and Maitra 1992, World Bank 1993). The initial models and estimates based on global standards concluded that the epidemic on the sub-continent of India could equal if not supersede that in Africa. This evidence was impossible to ignore partly since international agencies including the World Bank and the World Health Organization (WHO), bilateral development agencies such as USAID and DfID, and foundations such as the Ford Foundation had contributed extensively to funding and providing technical support to the health sector in India during the late 1980s and 1990s when evidence of HIV first emerged. The World Bank in particular was a strong partner through loans for infectious disease control and the WHO was a long-standing technical partner whose advice was taken seriously. In addition, many of these organisations offered funds, sponsored visits of senior government officials and parliamentarians to affected countries and provided technical support to a robust response to HIV, all of which was difficult to ignore. Most importantly, these partners provided global data on the raging epidemic in countries which had done little to address their HIV epidemics early on, and the consequential impact on their development indicators overall. This evidence bolstered the argument that India needed to act immediately and swiftly. It also provided evidence (limited though it was) of the steps that had helped slow down the epidemic in some countries despite an overall limitation of prevention, treatment and care options available at the time.

The action which needed to be taken far outstripped the Indian Government's expertise, experience and resources so, as a pragmatic approach, the government involved civil society in its AIDS response fairly early. There were rumblings among Indian civil society groups about concern for the growing epidemic in India among the people they served and the potential consequences of not acknowledging diversity in sexual identities and behaviours openly, not talking about sex and sexuality, and not addressing intolerant community norms around diverse sexual identities, behaviours and practices, especially in the context of mitigating stigma and discrimination. Some of these groups, such as Humsafar Trust working with gay men and Prerana and PSI India as well as the Sonagachi Project, working with and for sex workers and their clients, knew, understood and could approach at-risk populations on HIV prevention and care with a degree of mutual trust. In contrast, the government had a very limited relationship with at-risk populations whose behaviour was seen as 'immoral', 'illicit' and even un-Indian. Having civil society groups work directly with the at-risk populations thus kept the government at arm's length initially, which helped programmes to be more trusted and accepted by the populations they served but also served a pragmatic purpose initially with traditional elements of the populations who were still concerned about government attention towards so-far ignored populations. UNAIDS later documented the unusual approach that the Indian National AIDS Control Organization took of directly funding civil society groups through the procurement of their services (UNAIDS 2016) – a measure not taken earlier by the government, and involving community leaders, including those from at-risk and affected populations, in its advisory committees, contrary to the stigma and discrimination faced by these populations (Dube 2000).

The government also fostered inter-sectoral collaboration which led to the introduction of some of the potentially controversial but needed policies and programmes. The argument that HIV would erode the progress made in development indicators and make it even more difficult for India to rise as an economic power, captured the attention of finance, education and health ministries within government. Critical partners such as the media helped make the case eloquently, more persuasively and with larger outreach to the populace. The involvement of state-level politicians, technocrats, parliamentarians and ministers of health such as Shatrughan Sinha and Ambumani Ramadoss, who travelled to AIDS conferences and affected countries on visits funded by development partners and saw with their own eyes the ravages of the epidemic and the potential of a strong evidence-based and rights-informed response, made a difference. Some of these influencers subsequently worked with their constituencies to make a case for why it was imperative to introduce HIV prevention programmes, talk more about and ensure safe sex, and reduce the stigma and discrimination which drove HIV underground. And with time, they and their colleagues came to appreciate how India's development would be hampered if the epidemic was not contained, putting the lives of all its citizens at risk.

In addition to the evidence and the pragmatism underlying the response to HIV, a sound base of constitutional provisions established by the original writers of the Constitution of India, which promotes the protection of the weak, the poor and those who are marginalised, and the human rights treaties which India had ratified, strengthened the arguments for such a response. The legal community was quick to litigate against some of the early *faux pas* of the government in violation of the rights of those infected, using these very constitutional rights and going beyond them to argue for justice for all. Several seminal cases were fought and some won that fostered access to anti-retroviral drugs and overturned part of the Indian Penal Code criminalising sex between men. None of these outcomes would have been possible had India not already had in place the legal and constitutional protections that could be utilised, had it not committed itself to international human rights treaties, and had it not had a vibrant civil society which lobbied for justice in the face of a rapidly growing but still hidden epidemic. In pursuit of practical justice for all, forward-thinking members of the legal community joined hands with civil society and non-governmental organisations to bring these matters to the attention of the public and the courts, whether they succeeded in winning the relevant legal suits or not.

Of central importance, however, was the Indian Government's political understanding of what a massive AIDS epidemic might mean to India's future: the slowing down of development goals; the aid-related consequences of not taking heed of the covert warnings being given in case of inaction or faulty action, by its trusted partners; and international funding made available for the response. One of the covert factors which for instance triggered the interest of the Ministry of Finance was the reality of low foreign exchange levels, which made the potential influx of foreign exchange through a World Bank loan and other funding from international donors highly attractive. This aid came in various forms and through a variety of sources, but it also helped the government to use these funds partially to fix the weak and stretched health system, the limited capacity to gather reliable and sound data on health, and to integrate health issues across government departments and various sectors. Often unrecognised, and perhaps intentionally so, was the dynamic leadership shown by the administrative service officials collectively responsible at state and central levels for the HIV response. Many displayed a willingness to pick up the pace, to listen to divergent voices, especially civil society in all its manifestations including the media, along with health experts, both governmental and non-governmental, thereby promoting innovative methodologies to reach diverse populations. While none of this might seem revolutionary to some, these were not the standard approaches then taken by the Indian governmental machinery and they were unfamiliar in a climate where sex and sexuality were still taboo subjects. Rapid unlearning and learning helped lead the response, making it truly integrated, comprehensive and, as said earlier, informed by evidence, common sense and rights.

Legalisation of safe abortion in Mozambique

Overcoming cultural and historical barriers

Despite the fact that improvements in policies, programmes and practices have caused abortion to become safer the world over, a recent assessment worldwide indicates that most women continue to have only limited access to safe abortion (Barot 2018). A range of international human rights treaties, which most governments have ratified, support the right of a woman to liberty and to health (Center for Reproductive Rights 2017). Agreements such as the International Conference on Population and Development contain language that includes, at best, an obligation among governments to prevent unsafe abortion (UNFPA 2004), although not to make abortion legal.

The reality, however, is that abortion rights are the most contentious aspect of SRHR, despite evidence which shows several negative consequences, including higher rates of maternal mortality due to unsafe abortion (UNFPA 2004). Animosity towards access to contraception makes the situation even more complex since abortion is seen as equivalent to, or worse than, contraception, even though there is clear evidence to show that preventing unintended pregnancies through access to modern contraception reduces abortion rates (Bearak *et al.* 2018). One consequence of this is that if and where it is available, abortion is heavily regulated – such as being restricted to cases of rape and incest, where there is risk to the health of the mother, in the case of foetal abnormalities and available only through designated facilities and specific providers. The state-level restrictions in the USA have been described earlier. Stigma and discrimination surrounding abortion make the situation more complex, as well as barriers of physical access to abortion-providing clinics which sometimes are remotely located and few in number, or which have vigils outside the clinics by so-called 'pro-lifers' serving to enhance doubt and shame among prospective clients and offering a genuine threat to the safety of the clients and abortion providers, especially in the USA.

Access to contraception and safe abortion are particularly problematic in African countries, which collectively have the highest rates of mortality related to unsafe abortion (Guttmacher Institute 2018). And yet, abortion is heavily restricted, if available, in most African countries and legal in only five countries – Mozambique ranks among these five since 2014. The question is how this came to be in Mozambique.

Mozambique was ruled by Portuguese colonisers until 1975 and mired in civil war until 1992. As in many developing countries, women in Mozambique have always been particularly disadvantaged. UNICEF reports that more than 50 per cent of Mozambique women are illiterate, with high rates of school dropout, early marriage and lack of knowledge about birth-spacing among girls (UNICEF 2013). Mozambique has, however, bene-fited from strong leadership focusing on economic and social progress, but despite improvements overall, the total fertility rate in 2014 was 5.2 children per woman and the contraceptive prevalence rate was 11.6 per cent in 2011, ranking it 137 out of 147 countries worldwide, according to the World Health Organization (WHO 2015).

Mozambique also has one of the highest maternal mortality rates even today, despite a decline over the last decade. In 2008, the maternal mor-tality ratio was 550 per 100,000 live births, with many of the deaths being attributable to pregnancy or child birth-related complications due to abortion (WHO *et al.* 2010). The Millennium Development Goals (MDGs), to which all UN member states were signatory, included among its eight goals MDG goal 5 (to improve maternal health). Together, the MDGs pro-vided a motivation for countries, including those in Africa who were lagging behind in this goal, to contemplate bold action to accelerate pro-gress. The data from Mozambique and the push for reaching the MDGs provided incentive to Mozambique's political leadership to re-examine the issue of legal access to safe abortion through revision of the penal code, but what the government needed was an opportune moment to launch such action.

In 2003, acknowledging that Africa was lagging in maternal mortality and overall improvement of the status of women, the Assembly of the African Union developed the Maputo Protocol on the Rights of Women in Africa, which was signed by 46 of the 54 member states, including Mozambique. This Protocol upheld the right of women to control their fertility and access contraception in Article 14. In the appropriate measures mentioned in the Protocol that member states were expected to take to ensure these rights was included, 'authorizing medical abortion in cases of sexual assault, rape, incest and where the continued pregnancy endangers the mental and physical health of the mother or the life of the mother or the foetus' (African Union 2003). For Mozambique, this was an opportunity to revisit the issue of abortion, both to deliver on the Maputo commitment as well as to achieve its own development goals. The dominance of Catholicism and Islam among Mozambique's citizens had hitherto made abortion access a difficult issue. The Maputo Protocol provided both the impetus and moral argument, adding to the evidence, to take the issue seriously.

The Mozambique Government armed itself with evidence of the damage unsafe abortion was doing to its population and the inadequacy of the health system response, collected by the WHO, the national health system, and national and international experts (e.g. Gallo *et al.* 2004, Dgedge *et al.* 2005). It also adhered to the WHO guidance on safe abortion, which included law and policy reform as key measures (Hessini *et al.* 2006, WHO 2012). Political leadership in Mozambique post-independence was well informed around the issue. Pascoal Mocumbi, who was a medical professional with training in nursing and work experience in Mozambique as well as other African countries and those in the West (Ramsay 2003), had a strong background in this area and had made several attempts during his tenure as PM to experiment with greater access. His political background, having held several senior positions including prime minister in the mid-1990s until the mid-2000s, and his clout in the country helped give his views credibility.

Going a step further than the evidence, the government chose to involve its citizens in discussion around access to abortion. For instance, a public debate was launched on unsafe abortion, a multi-sectoral working group was set up to consider law reform, and an overhaul of the overall penal code (which had been inherited from the colonisers and never revised thereafter) was undertaken, which allowed abortion to be one of the issues addressed (Pathfinder International 2016). Extensive civil society engagement helped to keep the revision based on what would work in the context of the realities of different sections of society, especially women and the most vulnerable populations, and media engagement assisted in keeping the general population informed and involved in the evolution of the law.

Civil society engagement and public education were accelerated through the auspices of an existing network of civil society organisations, the Coalition for the Defence of Sexual and Reproductive Rights, which made abortion reform a near-exclusive focus of the Coalition from 2011 until 2014 when the abortion law was eventually passed (Pathfinder International 2016). A significant feature of this Coalition was its multi-disciplinary membership, constituting health groups, including those working on HIV, women's groups, young people's groups, and professional associations of medical, nursing and legal professionals. Prior to 2011, the Coalition had been working on a broader range of sexual and reproductive health issues and was a credible organisation which involved both local and international agencies with local presence. To ensure that its efforts around abortion were successful, the Coalition raised funds and developed a four-year strategic plan whose focus was public education, leadership education and media engagement around the need for a comprehensive law that permitted abortion under a broader set of conditions than earlier. It was quite successful in its goal in that the new law made legal abortion accessible on request (although restricted to officially designated facilities by 'qualified' practitioners) during the first 12 weeks of pregnancy in cases of physical or mental health consequences for the women, to 16 weeks in the case of incest and rape, and 24 weeks in cases of severe foetal abnormalities. The law also held the health sector responsible for creating these facilities and providing qualified practitioners.

Compared with the highly restrictive access to abortion permitted earlier, the new law was a major improvement and seen as a sign of success for the country and those who worked to make it happen.

Fostering change: lessons learned through the lens of practical justice

Looking at both these examples, one is struck by the complexity of the political, social and cultural contexts in which change occurred. When HIV was detected in India, there was trepidation that acknowledging the epidemic meant talking about sex and acknowledging the existence of behaviours and practices (which were stigmatised) such as sex work, drug use and sex between men, all of which were not the norm. Health, including sexually transmitted infections, had a very limited budget in the mid-1990s (Planning Commission of India 2009). For the Indian Government, it was not an easy decision to allocate large amounts of money to contain a growing but invisible epidemic, when the initial numbers were limited to specific populations who were marginalised, and when thousands more were affected by and died of other health conditions, such as tuberculosis, malaria and malnutrition (Vital Statistics Division, Office of the Registrar-General of India, Mortality Statistics of Causes of Death, New Delhi 1986, cited in Bhende and Kanitkar 1997). In the case of Mozambique, legalising abortion involved the complex process of changing the penal code and acknowledging publicly the existence of unsafe abortions. It also meant directly opposing the religious beliefs of the majority of the population and allocating fewer resources to other areas of need.

What is remarkable is that the changes which occurred had broader ramifications and were extensive. In the case of Mozambique, the legalisation of abortion under a wide range of conditions and for a longer period of time after conception was indeed a major gain in SRHR for the country. This benefited the maternal mortality rate, which, though still high, has gone down over time (WHO *et al.* 2010). For India, the change involved moving from an approach to HIV prevention by banning sex with foreigners and arguing that India's culture(s) would protect against HIV, to an approach of introducing family life (sex) education in schools, more open discussion about stigma and discrimination, the public involvement of people living with and affected by HIV in the response to HIV, the allocation of more resources to HIV, and most importantly, a much lower prevalence rate over time than expected. Today, while India still has the third-largest population of people living with HIV, the reported prevalence has fallen considerably to 0.26 per cent, with India achieving an overall reduction of 66 per cent in estimated annual new infections from 2000 (NACO 2015, UNAIDS 2017).

Looking at how the occurrence of change of this magnitude was accelerated from the practical justice lens, evidence stands out as important – both substantive, collected by reliable sources both national and international, as well as the sharing of personal experience, observations, testimonies and stories by those impacted. Denial and lack of knowledge are often at the root of societal indifference to the imperative for change. Making people, especially those in positions of influence, more aware of the scientific data and its implications for the development of the country played a central role. In the case of India, this evidence came from international health and development agencies and evidence from other developing countries at a more advanced stage of the epidemic. Together, these facilitated extrapolation to the Indian context in terms of what to do and what *not* to do if India wished to arrest the epidemic. Key parliamentarians' visits to other countries and their exposure to up-to-date evidence at international conferences had a more emotional impact, providing impetus for action. The media also provided public education and forums for debate and discussion around HIV. In the case of Mozambique, the evidence was more local in terms of the maternal mortality data as well as the unsafe abortion statistics, which kept Mozambique from reaching its development goals.

In both cases, civil society and media also held the government accountable for reaching its most marginalised and vulnerable populations to take appropriate action to mitigate the impact on their lives – there was evidence that these populations were suffering, and ignoring this suffering by the government was tantamount to not doing the right thing for its citizens. Pragmatically, and perhaps more importantly for some decision-makers, inaction would also slow down development and thereby impact the country as a whole.

Constitutionally, both the Indian and Mozambique governments were responsible for protecting their citizens, especially those most vulnerable (Government of India 2015, Government of Mozambique 2004). Being signatories to the major human rights treaties and conventions as well as less binding resolutions and internationally agreed development goals, governments were being held accountable for preserving the health and rights of the people so far as HIV and maternal mortality were concerned.

The right action in both instances was propelled by sound evidence which focused on the problem, the potential of an effective response, and the consequences of non-action or the wrong action. Also important was the sound normative argument advanced by credible and influential global, regional and national sources, building upon the commitments made by the governments to their peoples within the framework of the constitution and national legislation and agreed frameworks on human rights, health, and sexual and reproductive rights signed in the context of global forums such as the United Nations or regional fora such as the African Union.

Advocacy by civil society and the media also played a part in securing the positive outcomes described above. This helped foster multiple and hitherto unusual partnerships (such as that between civil society organisations and the government in the case of AIDS in India, and between media, civil society and government in the case of abortion in Mozambique), which helped shape the response to meet the needs of diverse sections of society. Smart strategies in presenting the change needed to different audiences appropriately, harnessing the momentum provided by international and regional policy initiatives in the case of Mozambique, and utilising the financial motivation offered by donors in the case of India enabled change to be accelerated.

Clearly these are but two moments in time when practical justice was served with admirable results. However, nothing remains static when it comes to change and the challenges to it. There is much that still needs to be done and there are often setbacks when it comes to change. In the case of India, investment in and attention to AIDS has dwindled recently, especially between 2014–15 and 2015–16, when it fell by 22 per cent (Agoramoorthy 2015). In the case of Mozambique, more research is needed to show whether the changes in law are being implemented so as to benefit the people since the maternal mortality rate has not yet dropped to the extent it should. Importantly, no magic formula exists for how desired change might best be brought about, especially since contextual specificity is so important. Nonetheless, if we are to plan for change in the current fractured and highly polarised climate around SRHR, we need to draw all the lessons we can from examples such as these, and approach change with a practical justice lens – and its commitment to sound evidence, good normative argument and the best mechanisms for achieving change within a particular context.

References

African Union, 2003. *Protocol to the African Charter on Human and Peoples' Rights on the Rights of Women in Africa.* Article 14, pp. 15–16. African Commission on Human and Peoples' Rights. Available from: www.achpr.org/instruments/women-protocol [Accessed 13 May 2018].

Agoramoorthy, G., 2015. India's Budget Reduction and AIDS Infections – Correspondence Piece. *The Lancet*, 15, June.

Barot, S., 2018. The Roadmap to Safe Abortion Worldwide: Lessons from New Global Trends on Incidence, Legality and Safety. *Guttmacher Policy Review*, 21, 17–22.

Bearak, J., Popinchalk, A., Alkema, L. and Sedgh, G., 2018. Global, Regional and Sub-regional Trends in Unintended Pregnancy and Its Outcomes from 1990 to 2014: Estimates from a Bayesian Hierarchical Model. *Lancet Global Health*, 6 (3), e380–e389.

Bhende, A. and Kanitkar, T., 1997. *Principles of Population Studies*. 10th edition. Mumbai: Himalaya Publishing House.

Carroll, A. and Mendos, L., 2017. *State Sponsored Homophobia 2017 Report: A World Survey of Sexual Orientation Laws: Criminalisation, Protection and Recognition*. Geneva: ILGA. Available from: www.ilga.org/downloads/2017/ILGA_State_Sponsored_ Homophobia_2017_WEB.pdf [Accessed 13 May 2018].

Center for Reproductive Rights, 2017. *The World's Abortion Laws*. New York: Center for Reproductive Rights. Available from: www.worldabortionlaws.com/ [Accessed 13 May 2018].

Dgedge, M., Gebreselassie, G., Bique, C., Victorino, M. T., Gallo, M F., Mitchell, E. M. H., King, K. O., Jamisse, L., Correa, D. M., de Almeida, E. and Chavane, L., 2005. *Confronting Maternal Mortality: The Status of Abortion Care in Public Health Facilities in Mozambique*. Chapel Hill, NC: Ipas.

Donovan, M. K., 2017. Postabortion Contraception: Emerging Opportunities and Barriers. *Guttmacher Policy Review*, 20 (2 October), 92–96. Available from: www. guttmacher.org/sites/default/files/article_files/gpr2009217.pdf [Accessed 2 May 2018].

Dube, S., 2000. *Sex, Lies and Drugs*. New Delhi: Harper Collins India.

Gallo, M., Gebreselassie, G., Victorino, M. T., Dgedge, M., Jamisse, L. and Bique, C., 2004. An Assessment of Abortion Services in Public Health Facilities in Mozambique: Women and Providers' Perspectives. *Reproductive Health Matters*, November, 12 (24 Suppl), 218–226.

Government of India, 2015. *The Constitution of India* [as on 9 November 2015]. New Delhi: Government of India, Ministry of Law and Justice (Legislative Department). Available from: www.india.gov.in/my-government/constitution-india/ constitution text [Accessed 13 May 2018].

Government of Mozambique, 2004. *The Constitution of Mozambique*. Available from: www.constituteproject.org/constitution/Mozambique_2007.pdf?lang=en [Accessed 13 May 2018].

Guttmacher Institute, 2017. *US Abortion Laws – Laws by State: An Overview of Abortion in the US*. New York: Guttmacher Institute. Available from: www.guttmacher.org/ fact-sheet/induced-abortion-worldwide [Accessed 13 May 2018].

Guttmacher Institute, 2018. *Fact Sheet: Abortion in Africa* [as at March 2018]. New York: Guttmacher Institute. Available from: www.guttmacher.org/sites/default/ files/factsheet/ib_aww-africa.pdf [Accessed 13 May 2018].

Hessini, L., Brookman-Amissah, E. and Crane, B., 2006. Global Policy Change and Women's Access to Safe Abortion: The Impact of the WHO's Guidance in Africa. *African Journal of Reproductive Health*, 10 (3), 14–27.

Mane, P. and Maitra, S., 1992. *AIDS Prevention: The Socio-cultural Context in India*. Mumbai: Tata Institute of Social Sciences.

NACO, 2015. *India HIV Estimations 2015: Technical Report*. New Delhi: NACO and National Institute of Medical Statistics, ICMR, Ministry of Health and Family Welfare.

Oronje, R., Crichton, J., Theobald, S., Lithur, N. O. and Ibisomi, L., 2011. Operationalising Sexual and Reproductive Health and Rights in Sub-Saharan Africa: Constraints, Dilemmas and Strategies. *BMC International Health and Human Rights*, 11 (Suppl 3), S8. doi: 10.1186/1472-698X-11-S3-S8.

Pathfinder International, 2016. *Strategies to Advance Abortion Rights and Access in Restrictive Settings: A Cross-country Analysis.* Watertown, MA: Pathfinder International.

Planning Commission of India, 2009. *National Health Accounts India, 2004–2005.* New Delhi: National Health Accounts Cell, Ministry of Health and Family Welfare.

Ramsay, S., 2003. Pascoal Mocumbi – International Health Advocate. *The Lancet,* 36 (9355). 400–403.

UNAIDS, 2016. *Governments Fund Communities: Six Country Responses of Financing Community Responses through Governmental Mechanisms.* Geneva: UNAIDS.

UNAIDS, 2017. *UNAIDS Data 2017.* Geneva: UNAIDS.

UNFPA, 2004. *Programme of Action Adopted at the International Conference on Population and Development, 5–13 September 1994.* New York: UNFPA.

UNICEF, 2013. *Mozambique Statistics.* Available from: www.unicef.org/infobycountry/mozambique_statistics.html [Accessed 13 May 2018].

WHO, 2012. *Safe Abortion: Technical and Policy Guidance for Health Systems on Safe Abortion.* Geneva: WHO.

WHO, 2015. *Mozambique Statistical Profile.* Geneva: WHO.

WHO, UNICEF, UNFPA and World Bank, 2010. *Trends in Maternal Mortality 1990–2008.* Geneva: WHO.

World Bank, 1993. *World Development Report 1993. Investing in Health, World Development Indicators.* New York: Oxford University Press.

Index

Page numbers in *italics* denote figures